Runner's World

STRENGTH TRAINING BOOK

Runner's World

STRENGTH TRAINING BOOK

by Edwin Sobey

Runner's World Books

Library of Congress Cataloging in Publication Data

Sobey, Edwin, J. C., 1948-
   Runner's world strength training book.

   1. Weightlifting. 2. Physical Fitness. 3. Exercise.
I. Title. II. Title: Strength training book.
III. Series
GV546.5.S6   796.4'1   81-8046
ISBN 0-89037-147-4 (spiral)   AACR2
ISBN 0-89037-238-1 (perfectbound)
ISBN 0-89037-249-7 (hardbound)

©1981 by
Edwin J.C. Sobey

New Edition 1982

No information in this book may be reprinted in any form
without permission from the publisher.
Runner's World Books
1400 Stierlin Rd.
Mountain View, CA 94043

Contents

Dedication. vi
Preface vii
Acknowledgments. viii
1. The Need for Strength Training. .1
2. Principles of Strength Training 11
3. Techniques 19
4. Aerobic Strength Training. 37
5. Strength Exercises. 49
6. Strength Programs for Sports .127
7. Strength Programs for Fitness. 155
8. Injuries 161
9. Strength Training for Women .171
    Bibliography 185
    About the Author. 187
    Recommended Reading. 189

Dedication

To
Barbara

Preface

Few people have been more predisposed against the use of weights than I once was. I knew the old myths berating weight lifting as truths and even correlated inversely weights pushed with intelligence. However, over the past six years I have gained an understanding and appreciation of what part strength training plays in fitness and in the preparation for sports.

This book was written for the many people who share my earlier views of weight or strength training. It will offer convincing proof that these people should try strength training, and will facilitate their first attempts if they do.

If you are one of those people who have never tried strength training, I urge you to commit yourself to a month-long program. At the end of the month if you find you do not like it, you probably never will like it—try some other form of exercise. But I believe that many people who try weight training will enjoy it and will stick with it as religiously as runners, swimmers, cyclists, or racquetball players follow their sports.

Do not approach weight training as a mindless exercise—clearly it is not. Besides deciding on a program and exercises, weight training tests the most basic mental powers—the powers to will mind over muscle. Merely going through the exercise motions workout after workout will not improve strength. Only by making yourself do more will you improve.

Also, approach the weight room as a place for social gatherings of people who share similar interests in strength and fitness. Workouts can and should be fun. If they were pure drudgery I would not have been doing them three days a week for the past six years. Make your workouts fun—as well as physically rewarding.

Acknowledgments

With the greatest appreciation I acknowledge the contributions of Vicki Crawford, who typed the manuscript; Marina Ossipov, who prepared the illustrations; Marsha Burch who wrote Chapter 9, and Suzie Eitel, who reviewed the manuscript.

Special thanks goes to James Wiltjer, vice president of the Los Altos Health Club in Los Altos, California, for making available the club's facilities. The author would also like to thank Peter Lehner, an instructor at Los Altos Health Club, for his tireless efforts lifting weights in front of the camera of Jeff Reinking.

1

The Need for Strength Training

> "....research generally demonstrates that specific sports skills such as speed in running, swimming, throwing.... and jumping all can be improved significantly through weight training programs."
>
> —Mathews and Fox

Over the last decade a large number of Americans have become involved in sports and physical fitness. Attitudes have been changing—sports are no longer only for the young, and physical fitness has become a way of life for many of us.

Cardiovascular-respiratory fitness is the locker room battle cry. People are running, swimming, cycling, skiing, or hiking. Often they take up these activities initially for fitness, but with time they begin pursuing them primarily for the enjoyment. But to be physically fit or to do well in a sport or to enjoy a physical activity requires attention to flexibility and strength. Few people who start fitness programs or who engage in sports are inherently interested in improving their flexibility. Many of them have learned, however, that in order to continue the active life a stretching program was called for. Stretching brings increased flexibility, which is needed for many activities and helps prevent injuries. Also, it has been shown that an improvement in athletic performance can be the result of improved flexibility; now stretching is an integral part of most fitness or sports programs.

But strength conditioning has been overlooked largely because of myths and misunderstandings about its objectives and results. Watching the superheavy weight lifters in the Olympics or body-building contests only encourages the popular impression that being strong means being large and abnormally shaped.

This book does not deal with competitive weight lifting or body building. Our subject is strength training. The purpose of strength training is to achieve an optimum level of strength fitness or to improve performance in a sport or physical activity through the use of weights.

Since the word strength appears in the title and throughout this book, a definition is required. By strength, we mean muscular strength. Muscular strength is the force a muscle can exert. When we speak of muscular endurance, we mean strength, or muscle force, exerted over a long period of time. Power is the rate of speed at which a force can be exerted. Strength, power and endurance all describe the force a muscle can exert. Often power is used to describe the application of strength over a short span of time. In this connotation, power and endurance have opposite meanings: power means sudden bursts of strength, and endurance means prolonged exertions of strength. The differences between the two terms are based on the element of time—how many muscle contractions can you do, how long can you keep contracting a muscle, or how fast can you contract a muscle against a given resistance.

Strength refers to an absolute measure of muscular force. More important is a measure of a person's strength fitness. If I can bench press 50 pounds more than you can, it does not mean that I have a higher degree of strength fitness. Strength fitness refers to the optimal level of strength that an individual needs and wants, to perform whatever activity he or she desires. Strength fitness should be the goal, not pure strength.

Although strength training can help to improve performance in almost any physical endeavor, continuously increasing strength will not necessarily cause continued improvement in performance. Too much strength can even have a negative effect, causing a deterioration in performance. The runner who unnecessarily increases his muscle mass beyond optimum levels lowers his running performance because he carries extra weight. He may well be the strongest man in the race, but he probably will not be the fastest man. Furthermore, strength training for a sport takes time and energy that could be spent on training skills for the sport. An exclusive training regime consisting of building strength instead of practicing your sport or event will invariably result in a poor performance.

Your goals for strength fitness will and should change as you learn more about strength and about your body. Several studies have shown that improvements in performance occur from strength training but few studies describe optimal techniques for individual sports. Thus, you will need to experiment to find the optimal levels of strength and the optimal programs to maximize performance in your sport.

Strength training is also individualistic. There are a few well-accepted principles (these are explained in Chapter 2) and an endless supply of ideas and theories. You must sort through the ideas and theories and use the ones that work for you. To be effective, your training program should have (at least general) goals. To meet these goals you need to experiment with techniques and schedules. This book will give you the information you need to establish and meet your goals.

BENEFITS OF STRENGTH TRAINING

Obviously, without strength there can be no movement. Some minimum level of strength is needed for every physical activity. In many activities performance can be increased more dramatically with the addition of strength development in the training program than with any other form of training. In any sport an athlete's performance is limited to his or her weakest link. The middle-distance runner who does not have the strength to kick or to accelerate during the last 200 yards may lose. His endurance may have been the best in the field, he may have great flexibility and good running form, but still lose. Even a modest strength training program could quickly (within three to six weeks) and efficiently (less than two hours a week) improve his kick. It probably would also improve his stride and running form. Most sports require a higher level of strength than running does. But even running can improve with strength training.

There is a continuing debate among running coaches about the merit of strength-training programs for long-distance runners. For sprinters and middle-distance runners, strength training is universally accepted. Sebastian Coe, current world-record holder in the 800-meter, and former record holder in the 1500-meter and mile is a strong advocate of strength training, especially aerobic strength training (see Chapter 4). But for the higher endurance races, the renowned coach Arthur Lydiard of New Zealand believes strength

4 THE NEED FOR STRENGTH TRAINING

training only robs runners of time and energy that should be spent in running. The late Percy Cerutty would have disagreed and pointed as evidence to a number of champion long-distance runners who lifted weights. If you are a long-distance runner you must face this question yourself. If you compete, try weight training and see if you like the results. For non-competitive runners, strength training, along with flexibility training, will complete your fitness program.

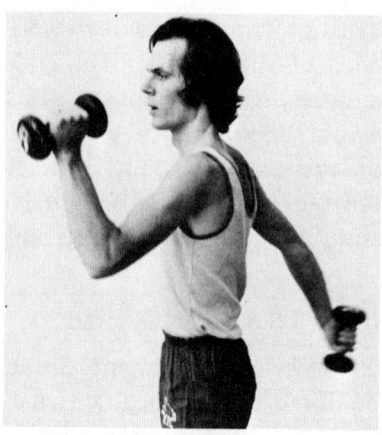

Weightlifters have quick relfexes.

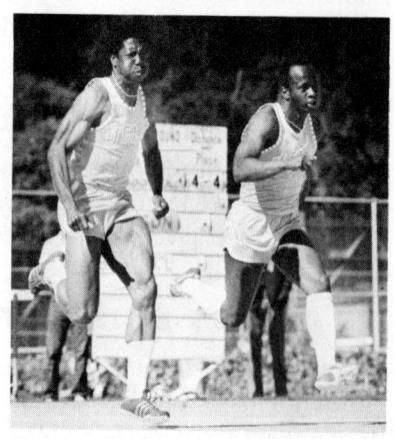

Sprinters have overspecialized leg muscles.

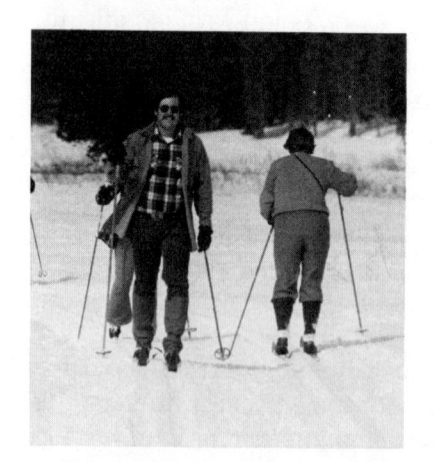

Cross-country skiers use strength training to build endurance.

In most other sports, acceptance of strength training is growing. Doc Counsilman advocates a dry-land strength program for swimmers. Art Dickinson (advisor to the U.S. Olympic ski team) suggests that even recreational cross-country skiers in addition to competitive skiers should weight train. In sports such as football, where strength is very important, weight training is an integral part of the workouts.

In almost every sport some muscles are used more than their antagonists. This imbalance is especially true in running. The overspecialization of muscles, or the development of a muscle, for only one motion and the lack of development for its antagonist, can cause problems for the athlete. Sprinters have a high occurrence of hamstring pulls partly because the hamstring is much weaker than its antagonist, the quadricep. Thus the athlete should ensure an optimum ratio of strength between the prime muscles needed for his sport and the opposing muscles. For the person interested just in fitness, and not in competition, the development of strength balance between antagonists should be a goal of his fitness program. For each exercise performed, there should be another exercise for the antagonists. If the strength-training program does not include exercises for both sets of opposing muscles, the strength imbalance will manifest itself in poor posture or muscle injuries.

Strength training improves muscle strength but also improves muscle endurance and speed. Having muscle endurance means that a person has the strength to overcome some force or resistance many times, or to hold a given position for a long time. Experiments have shown a high correlation between strength gains and improvements in muscle endurance. The stronger a muscle is, the less relative effort it must exert to overcome the force. A weak muscle may be taxed to near maximal effort to perform each contraction while a stronger muscle will operate at a submaximal level. Thus the stronger muscle will not fatigue as quickly as the weak one.

The speed of muscle contraction also is increased through strength training. This is counter to what most people expect. Weight lifters have faster reflexes than most other athletes (including race-car drivers). The increase in speed with strength is probably a neurological response to the repetitive training. By doing the same motions over and over, the body learns to do the motion more effectively. The stimulation of muscles by nerves is improved by increasing the number of nerve motor units.

There is another neurological aspect of improved speed. In order to move, one muscle must shorten and its antagonist must lengthen. Nerve impulses must be sent to both muscles, telling one to contract and the other to relax. This coordination of muscles can be improved through strength training.

Improving speed improves the power a muscle can develop. Power is the product of strength and speed. Only in a few events is strength alone the desired trait. Usually in "strength events" the speed at which the muscle can be contracted is as important as strength. Improving power, not just strength, therefore should be the goal in preparation for such events. Since strength training can improve both strength and speed, it is fully applicable.

An important but often overlooked aspect of strength development is the improvement in self-confidence. Watching yourself improve and seeing that you can do today what you could not have done only a few weeks ago provides a sense of accomplishment. Also, knowing how hard you can push your body in the weight room gives you confidence to push yourself equally hard in other activities. This is especially true for older women who have not had a background of organized sports. They are reluctant to push themselves or to experience the pain of muscle exertion. A progressive resistance program along with positive encouragement can help them gain strength and to achieve their athletic potential.

The improvement in self-confidence provides a positive feedback to strength training. Once you have developed a new mental image of yourself, you expect to and make special sacrifices to maintain it. You will not allow yourself to lose the strength you have gained. Instead of taking it easy in your workouts you will push yourself to improve, because you have grown to expect that.

Another benefit of strength training is improved joint stability. Injuries to knees and ankles, and to a lesser degree hips, are a common occurrence in many sports. Strength training is recommended for preventing these injuries and for rehabilitating injuries. When an exercise is performed over a long period of time with a progressively larger exercise resistance, the muscles and connective tissues thicken. This stabilizes the joint and protects it from overuse injuries or from impact injuries. Physical therapy for injuries around joints focuses on the development of muscles to rehabilitate the patient and to prevent reccurrence of the injury.

As you get older, strength training should become more important. With increasing age, beyond 30 years, muscles tend to atrophy or get smaller. To keep up the same level of activity as you get older this process must be reversed or at least stopped. A well-conceived strength training program can do that.

It is nice to know that once you have improved your strength it will deteriorate at a slow rate. While three workouts a week are recommended to improve strength, only one a week is needed to maintain that strength. Even if training is stopped altogether, the decrease in strength is slow. In one experiment, subjects trained for twelve weeks and then stopped. One year later they were tested and researchers found that the subjects had retained 45 percent of the strength gained in the 12-week training period. In another experiment it was found that a significant amount of strength developed in the experimental program was retained even after 18 months without strength training. We do not recommend this kind of training schedule, but it is nice to learn that your investment in strength training pays dividends over a long period. It is also nice to know that strength gains can occur much more quickly than the process of decay.

If you do stop your strength-training program and then restart it, you will find it much easier to regain your previous levels of strength than it was initially. One study found that it took only one-fourth the number of training sessions to regain the previous strength level. Once a good base of muscle tone is developed, deterioration by neglect will go slowly. Even a modest training program will maintain strength. This point is important to remember in scheduling a year-round training program for a particular sport. Levels of strength built in the off-season can be maintained during the preseason with occasional workouts. Strength workouts can even be stopped altogether during the competitive season with little loss in strength. Thus as the competitive season approaches, more training effort can be devoted to the specific skills of the sport while maintaining the strength gained in the off-season.

DISPELLING THE MYTHS

Although more and more people have started fitness programs over the past few years, most have avoided strength training. This is due, at least in part, to the prevailing stereotypes of strength trainers and to misconceptions about the purpose and results of strength development. Here are some myths and truths.

Strength training adds bulk. This is partially true. There is an increase in muscle mass as a result of training; however, the increase is usually small and is accompanied by a loss of fat. Experiments have found little or no change in total body weight following a strength-training program. However, they report a significant loss in body fat and a significant gain in lean body weight.

The increase in muscle mass is fairly small, especially for women. The outrageous musculature of body-builders does not come from a simple strength program. Their goal is to add muscle mass. In most sports, added mass is not an asset and is often a liability. If you want to bulk up for the beach or body-building contests this book is not for you.

Many women avoid strength training for fear of developing large or unsightly bulges. This does not happen. Only about 5 percent of the population of women will significantly increase their muscle mass. Any increase in muscle mass will be much smaller one tenth as much for women than for men on identical programs. In one experiment, the largest increase in muscle size for women was less than a quarter-inch. The difference in ability between men and women to add muscle mass, or to hypertrophy, is due to the male hormone testosterone. Testosterone regulates hypertrophy. The relatively high levels of this hormone in men (very low in women) allow them to easily increase muscle size while very few women can. However, this does not mean that women do not gain strength from training—they certainly do, but usually without a significant increase in muscle mass.

Although we do not advocate strength training as a beauty aid for women, it can improve figures. Muscles become firmer, although not bigger, and posture improves. Body fat is lowered, especially around hips, thighs and buttocks. Ladies, do not let pictures of East German women shot-putters keep you away from strength training.

There are four principal changes that occur when strength is imposed. There can be an increase in the size (diameter) of the muscle fibers that make up a muscle. These fibers are small, ranging in diameter from 1/1000 of a centimeter (a centimeter is about 4/10 of an inch) to 1/100 of a centimeter. The diameter of a fiber correlates with the work-load that is usually imposed on the muscle.

Along with the increase in fiber size comes an increase in the amount of protein in the muscle. Muscle is composed of about 20 percent protein (and 75 percent water) and so any increase in size is accompanied by increased quantities of protein.

The density of capillaries in the muscle increases, allowing oxygen in the blood to be brought to the muscle more efficiently and waste products of the muscle to be carried away quicker. Both of these processes help prevent muscle fatigue.

Also, accompanying strength gains are increases in amounts of connective tendinous and ligamentous tissues. As these tissues thicken, the chance of injuring the muscle or the joint that is supported is reduced.

You can significantly increase your muscle mass through strength training if you follow fairly specific body-building rules. This is, however, not the objective of the programs described in this book. There will be some increase in muscle size with strength training but it will not be noticeable for women and only slightly so for most men. The amount of increase is determined largely by your genetics.

Strong people are muscle-bound. Muscle-boundness, or lack of flexibility can come about as the result of improper training. However, a properly designed program will probably improve flexibility. The key here is to make muscle flexibility one of the goals of a fitness or sports preparation program. With an adequate stretching regime, if you develop strength through the full range of motion you will not lose flexibility.

Reflex speed decreases with strength. As mentioned above, this is simply not true. Just the opposite occurs; speed increases with strength improvement. This myth probably began with the stereotype of the muscle-bound weightlifter whose muscles were so ponderous that it took several seconds to move them. Experiments have shown, however, that reflex speed becomes faster as strength is improved, probably because an increase in nerve-muscle activation units accompanies strength gains.

When you stop training, muscle turns to flab. Muscle is protein and water and no alchemy yet known can turn that into fat. Muscles hypertrophy, or grow, when they are subjected to work and they atrophy, or get smaller, when they are not worked. Fat is stored in the body when the calories consumed exceed the calories used to perform work. The two equations are independent. If you stop training, your muscles will slowly lose strength and will atrophy. Your weight may go up if you consume the same quantities of food and beverage that you did while training. If you cut back on training, you should also cut back on your caloric intake.

Strength training is just for men. Like many myths, this one is in direct opposition to the facts. Men typically have a higher state of strength development than women. Therefore, women have more potential to benefit from strength training.

Improvement in sports is more strength-limited for women. Men often have the required strength and need to develop technique. Women lack the strength and must refine their techniques to a higher degree to achieve the same results. Even a few weeks of strength training can bring phenomenal improvements. I witnessed this after I developed a strength program for young women gymnasts. After two weeks in a very modest program they were able to execute moves and perform gymnastic exercises that they had been trying to do for months.

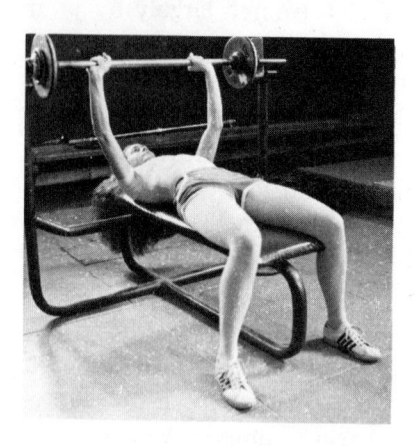

Strength training is for women, too.

For women who compete in endurance events, strength training may be more beneficial than for men in the same events. Women can gain strength and be almost assured that their body weight will not increase. Some men add bulk easily and thus must balance their strength gain against the negative aspects of gaining weight.

The development of strength is as important to women as to men. While the iron-pumping crowd may think that the weight room is the last bastion of masculinity, women's dues and their facility-fee payments are also helping to pay for the equipment.

2

Principles of Strength Training

To strengthen a muscle it "should be subjected to strenuous exercise and, at regular intervals, to maximum exertion."

—De Lorme

There are many ideas on how to gain strength efficiently. Unfortunately most of these ideas have not been adequately tested in controlled experiments. There are, however, two principles that have stood the test of time and have become universally accepted. Understanding these principles is fundamental to developing a strength-training program.

SPECIFIC ADAPTATION TO IMPROVE DEMANDS

This is also called the specificity principle. It refers to the fact that the body adapts so that it can most easily perform the work usually expected of it. If preparing for a marathon, you would not train by playing football. You might get a good cardiovascular workout, but the training effects would not transfer—that is, they would not be of much use in distance racing. Thus, most training should be specific to the sport in which you want to compete.

In strength training for sports you need to ascertain what motions are performed, at which speeds and what muscles are involved, then design a program to strengthen these muscles. The strength you develop will be specific to the exercise performed. Doing pushups is no help in preparation for doing pull-ups. Your strength-training program must be geared to developing useful strength and your exercises should closely mimic the particular movements in your sport.

An exercise performed through a limited range of motion will develop strength only through that same range. Strength at one position is not transferable to other positions. Thus if you use isometric exercises (exercises that do not involve movement—strength is exerted against immovable objects) you must do them several times at different angles to develop strength through a range of motion. Strength development is specific (or limited) to the angle at which an exercise is performed.

A common mistake in strength training is to do an exercise through a restricted range of motion in order to do more repetitions. When doing a pushup it is relatively easy to move up and down a few inches without getting one's chest to the floor. Because they can do more pushups this way, people mistakenly believe they are getting a better workout. To develop strength throughout the range of motion you must exercise through the full range of motion.

Exercising through the full ranges has an additional benefit: maintenance of flexibility. Muscles shorten and tighten if worked through a limited range. Without corrective action this can lead to being muscle-bound.

The speed of movement in your sport is also specific to the work load imposed on a muscle. If you are training for a speed event, you need to perform fast repetitions. You must also ensure that the movement you need to perform in your sport is duplicated as closely as possible in your training. The speed that you develop in training is specific to the limit that is exercised and even to the particular direction of motion of the exercise.

An additional point needs to be made. Actions in almost every sport require contractions of many muscles; however, in training for strength it is most efficient to isolate individual muscles as much as possible. Isolation means that only one muscle performs an exercise. When a muscle is isolated it can be overloaded (or worked beyond what it's used to) which causes rapid gains in strength. When several sets of muscles are used to perform an exercise, the larger muscles do most of the work. This ensures that the smaller muscles do not get a good workout, and the exercise is usually too easy for the larger muscles, so they also lose out.

Principles of Strength Training 13

A good example of the importance of isolation is the military or standing press. This is an exercise for arms and shoulders. How-

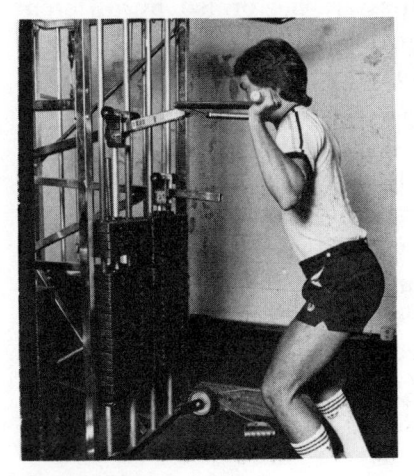

The standing military press.   This isolates arms and shoulders.

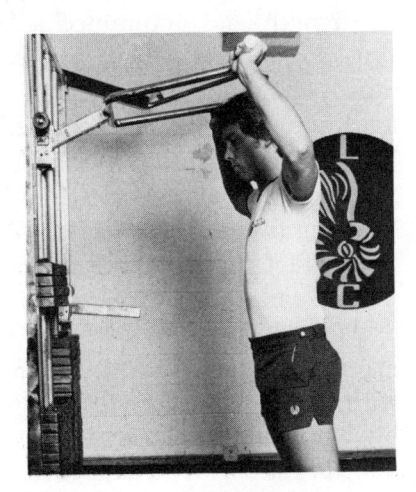

ever, as these muscles become tired there is a tendency to bend the back, knees or hips. These much larger muscles are contracted quickly to accelerate the weight upward in order to take some of the burden from the arms and shoulders. The weight used for this exercise is too light to cause any strength gain in the larger muscles. Since the last few repetitions of an exercise are the most important, the arm and shoulder muscles are being robbed of their training by the undesirable assistance. Thus it is important to ensure that each exercise is performed correctly and that only the muscles being exercised are used.

There is a conflict between isolating a muscle to develop strength and duplicating sports movements that may require several muscles working together. The way out of this dilemma is to use two methods of training: develop a good level of muscle strength (isolation training) during the off-season and mimic sports movements in preseason training. Since strength decays at a slow rate, the isolation training will provide the strength needed throughout the sport's season (see Chapter 6 for details of scheduling strength training throughout the year).

During the preseason, strength training should mimic not only the action involved in a sport but also the speed of contraction. Sports that involve fast motion require rapid movement in training. Those that involve endurance require many repetitions in training.

Remember that the changes that take place in a muscle as a result of training are specific to the type of exercise.

Strength and endurance activities are performed by different types of muscle fibers. There are three types of muscle fibers. Slow-twitch fibers are rich in capillaries; they fatigue slowly and are responsible for success in endurance events. Fast-twitch fibers have a lower density of capillaries; they fatigue quickly but provide a high level of strength quickly. Recently a third muscle type has been found—a fast-twitch fiber that's fatigue-resistant.

The fact that everyone is endowed with a different proportion of fast-and slow-twitch fibers partly explains why most people excel at some sports and fail at others. Frank Shorter, the Olympic marathoner, played football in secondary school. Had he stayed with it rather than switching to cross-country and track he probably would not be the well-known athlete he is today. Undoubtedly Shorter is a slow-twitch man.

In a pamphlet entitled "Endurance Training for the Elite Runner," Professor Pat O'Shea lists the relative percentages of fast- and slow-twitch fibers among successful athletes.

Sport	Percentage Fast-twitch	Slow-twitch
Olympic weightlifters	83	17
Sprinters	78	22
Downhill skiers	52	48
Marathon runners	26	74

Although athletic training probably cannot change the proportions of fast- and slow-twitch fibers, it can selectively increase the work capacity of one or the other.

The important point here is that to be successful an athlete needs to achieve some proportion of slow- and fast-twitch fibers that is specific to his sport. His genetic inheritance exerts control over the proportion. However, training can emphasize the development of one or the other, and thus it should be geared toward developing the type of muscle fiber needed for the sport.

THE OVERLOAD PRINCIPLE

For a muscle to gain strength it must be overloaded. That is, it must be required to do more than it is used to doing. To determine if a muscle is overloaded, a chart is shown comparing work accomplished and plotted against exercise resistance. Work is the

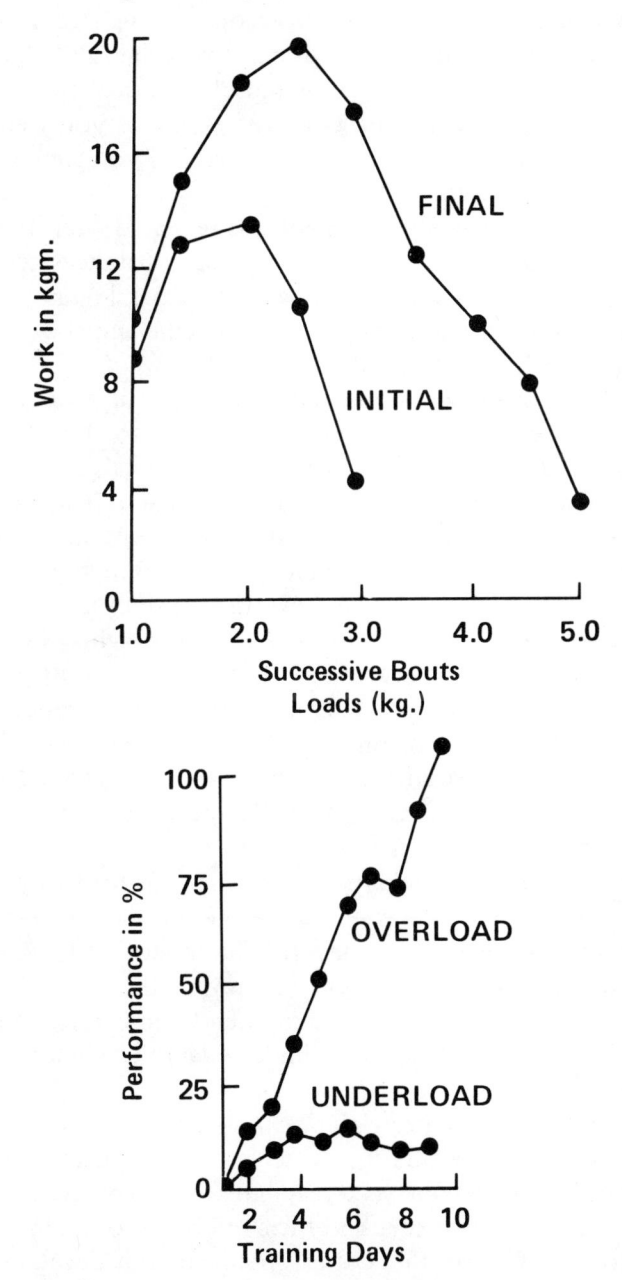

Reprinted from *Physical Therapy* (vol. 36: pp. 371-383, 1956) with the permission of the American Physical Therapy Association.

product of weight, repetition, and distance moved. The idea is to determine at what weight a particular muscle can perform the most work in a limited time. In the accompanying figure the maximum work occurred at two kilograms during the first experiment. Using an exercise resistance for the muscle less than two kilograms would not cause a significant gain in strength. If you were to use this curve to pick the weight for an exercise, you should choose either two kilograms or slightly higher.

Notice that when the experiment was repeated later, there were increases in work capacity at all exercise resistances tested and that the overload point moved upward to 2.5 kilograms. To continue improving strength, the exercise resistance must be increased to keep the muscle overloaded.

In strength training, the exercise resistance or weight must be larger than the muscle has become adapted to. Using a lighter weight or smaller resistance will result in minimal, if any, gains in strength. This point is shown in the next figure. The two curves represent two groups of people engaged in an experiment to evaluate strength improvement techniques. The group represented by the upper curve used weights that overloaded their muscles. People represented in the lower curve used lighter weights. Each group did the same amount of work in training. The group using the lighter weights (not overloaded) did more sets of repetitions so that the work load was the same.

The difference in results is phenomenal. The overloaded group achieved large gains in strength while the other group achieved essentially none.

This is important in evaluating strength needs for various sports. For example, in distance running the muscles in the upper body are never overloaded. They may tire or fatigue but running will not cause them to get stronger. To prevent them from fatiguing in a long race the runner must strengthen them through a progressive overload exercise program. Similar examples abound in other sports.

When exercise resistance is chosen so that the muscle is overloaded, the muscle will fatigue after a few repetitions. The first one or two repetitions may be easy but with each additional repetition the muscles tire more and the exercise becomes increasingly harder to do. This is the critical point to the development of strength. It is not the first few repetitions that cause strength gains, it is the last one or two. Here is where determination and self-discipline become important. It is easy to quit when the exercise gets tough. But the muscle must be pushed toward the point where it will no longer respond.

As gains in strength are made, the exercise resistance must be progressively increased. Progressive overloading is a fundamental technique for strength training. As a muscle adapts by growing stronger, heavier loads are placed on it. When the resistance is not progressively increased it will soon be too light, the muscle will no longer be overloaded, and no gains in strength will occur.

For best results in strength training, the exercise resistance must be gradually increased over a long period of time. The demands imposed on a muscle cannot be increased quickly. It takes time for muscles to grow and adapt and it is important not to strain them. The old adage "train, don't strain" is important to remember.

When you overload your muscles, you must give them the chance to rest from workouts. Training every day will not allow the muscles time to recuperate and strength will actually decrease. (The exception to this rule is a "split routine." See Chapter 3). Training once a week is not often enough. The benefits of the last workout will have been largely lost before the next session occurs. Two or three days after a workout, strength levels start to decline. To make progress you must work out again before a significant loss in strength occurs, but after an adequate period of rest. The optimum schedule seems to be three times a week on non-consecutive days. An alternate schedule is to work out every other day.

When starting a strength-training program using the overload principle, you will achieve large increases in strength quickly. Typical results are between 5- and 12-percent gains in strength per week. At these rates you would double your strength every six to 12 weeks. Unfortunately, this will not occur. As you get stronger it will take increasingly more effort to gain strength. The law of diminishing returns creeps in as it does in any training program. To continue to improve your strength you will need to devote more time and energy to your training. Obviously there comes a point at which either you become satisfied with your level of strength or eventually your body rebels and falls victim to injury.

Gains in strength do not occur at an even pace. As mentioned previously, large gains are made early in a program. Then you

18   PRINCIPLES OF STRENGTH TRAINING

reach a plateau; training can be discouraging as you exert a large effort but see little or no gain. But plateaus can be broken through (see Chapter 3) and then relatively rapid increases in strength occur again. But as you continue to train, the plateaus come closer together, and strength gains are smaller. By this point you are approaching your maximum potential.

In preparation for your season it is desirable to be near your peak before preseason training begins. The pre-preseason training occurs in what used to be the offseason. During the preseason you should attempt to transfer the strength you have gained into the motions of your sport.

3

Techniques

"....mere repetition of contractions which place no stress on the neuromuscular system has little effect on the functional capacity of the skeletal muscles."
—Hellebrandt and Hartz

EXERCISE TYPES

There are three methods of developing strength. They are classified on the basis of holding constant speed, resistance or position. The three methods are called isokinetic, isotonic and isometric.

Isometrics enjoyed a period of popularity a few years ago in this country. They were touted as being an easy and fast way to build strength. Their rapid demise suggests that isometrics are neither fast nor easy.

The word isometrics means that the length of a muscle being exercised does not change during the exercise. Standing in a doorway and pushing outward against the door frame on both sides is an example of an isometric exercise. Since no elaborate equipment is needed to do isometrics, they can be performed anywhere. For a person who sits most of the working day, isometrics are a good method of exercising muscles while at a desk.

We do not advocate isometrics for an active training program. Although it is difficult to compare results between the different exercise types, it appears that isometrics is the least efficient method of developing strength. Also, with isometrics there is little or no increase in the speed of contraction, whereas significant gains can be achieved with both of the other methods. The rate of

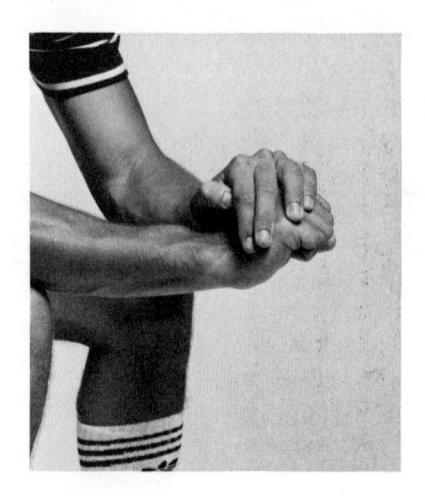

Isometrics can be done anywhere.

progress is difficult to gauge with isometrics since there is no movement. With the other methods, exercise resistance and the number of repetitions can be monitored. Seeing progress is an important incentive in training. It is easy to lose interest in isometrics, where no progress is measured.

The one advantage isometrics have is that they are fast. Muscles are contracted for only a few seconds. However, because strength gains are specific to the angle of exercise, isometric exercises must be repeated at several different angles. This robs them of much of their touted advantage for saving time.

Isotonics are the type of exercise usually associated with strength training. The weight or exercise resistance is constant throughout a repetition. Examples of isotonic exercises are pushups or working with dumbbells.

With isotonics, muscle strength can be developed while the muscle is either contracting or lengthening. The former, called concentric exercising, is by far the more popular. Eccentric exercising, also called negative exercising or negative lifting, is done while the muscle is lengthening.

Any exercise that can be done concentrically can be done eccentrically. Instead of overcoming the gravitational force of exercise weights, the force is increased until it is greater than the force a muscle can deliver. Instead of pumping weights upward against gravity, the weights are increased and the exerciser tries to resist the downward movement of the weights. Obviously some assistance is needed in raising the weights up to their initial position

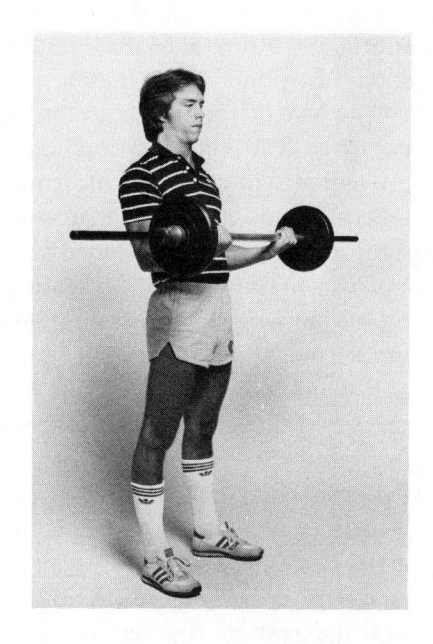

Arm curls are isotonic exercise.

for the next repetition. Assistance is also needed to ensure that the person exercising does not lose control of the weights.

The theory behind negative lifting is that since larger weights can be used, a faster progression of strength can be obtained. Since it requires assistance of at least one spotter at each station and since its effectiveness is unknown, negative lifting is not generally recommended. Throughout the rest of this book when we refer to isotonics we mean concentric exercising.

It is difficult to compare the effectiveness of isometrics and isotonics because it is hard not to bias the test. How does one measure strength gain except by an isometric or isotonic test? A group trained on isometrics would seem to have a specific advantage if the test were isometric, but a surprising result of one comparison was that isotonically trained subjects showed greater strength gains on isometric tests than did isometrically trained subjects. This one test does not imply that isotonics are necessarily always a better method. However, it does suggest that isotonics may be a more efficient method of strength training.

There are other advantages of isotonics over isometrics. Speed and endurance training can be performed with isotonics but not with isometrics. Improvements in motor ability accompany isotonic strength gains but are seen in isometrics only to a small degree; furthermore, it seems logical to assume that since most sports or other activities require isotonic contractions, training should be done in this manner.

The last difference between isometrics and isotonics is the most important. It is motivation. Using isotonics enables you to see improvements in strength: more repetitions can be done or larger resistances can be used. Each success or improvement provides motivation for future improvements. If, however, you prefer isometrics and can maintain the motivation to continue training with them, then you will be successful. Motivation is more fundamental to success in strength training than the particular method employed.

Isotonic methods have one major drawback. Although the exercise resistance is constant throughout an exercise, the difficulty the muscle overcomes varies greatly. As an example, picture the two-arm curl with a barbell. Moving the barbell initially is easy because much of the movement is parallel to the floor and there is little movement upward, against gravity. If the weight is accelerated very quickly here, the biceps will do little or no work throughout the rest of the repetition. In this case the weight has been thrown upward, not lifted. This is called the ballistic effect. Any extraneous movement in the legs, hips, or back will further accelerate the weight so that the biceps are getting no exercise at all.

Even if the barbell were not unduly accelerated initially, the force needed to move it varies. Initially, as stated above, the force is small. The force is at a maximum when the forearm and upper arm are at a 90-degree angle. Here movement is nearly vertical and is directly opposed by gravity.

The importance of the variance in force in an exercise is that the strength gained by the muscle is specific to the angle at which force was applied. A force unevenly distributed throughout the repetition will cause uneven gains in strength. The largest gains will occur where the resistance is greatest. Further, since the maximum weight that can be lifted on any repetition is limited to the maximum that can be handled in the weakest part of the repetition, efficient strength gains can only occur at that one spot.

The weakest angle of an exercise is called the sticking point. Until strength is improved here, you cannot increase the exercise resistance and, thus, at other angles of the motion the muscle may be underloaded.

One way to overcome this difficulty is to mechanically adjust the exercise resistance on weight machines so that the effective load is held constant throughout the exercise. This equalizes the force the muscle exerts throughout the range of motion—there are no sticking points. Elaborate equipment to do this has been designed and is becoming popular among strength trainers. These

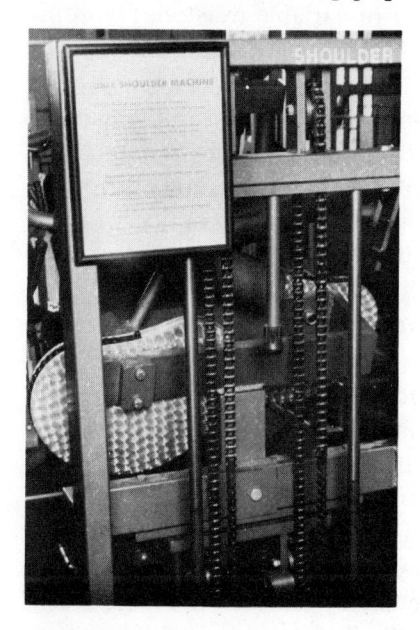

Nautilus equipment is variable-resistance isotonic.

machines, sold as Nautilus and Dyna cam, and others, are classified as variable-resistance isotonic. Unsubstantiated claims by manufacturers to the contrary, there is little evidence to suggest that this method is more efficient for strength training.

There are two factors to consider in using the variable-resistance equipment. Many of the manufacturers of this equipment have gone to great lengths to isolate the particular muscles being exercised. To do this effectively, they have designed equipment with variable seating heights, safety belts, and complicated movements. The benefit to this is that it is much harder to cheat while doing arm exercises—that is when you are doing an arm exercise, for example, it is difficult to cheat by using back or leg motion to overcome the sticking point. By better isolating a muscle you can get faster gains in strength development because the resistance is concentrated on the particular muscle. Unfortunately, few sports activities are similar to the artificial movements used in these exercises. In training for most sports you could not achieve specific movements similar to your sport with any machine, especially these. Also, since many motions in sports are ballistic in nature, it makes sense to use ballistic motion in training. Removal of the ballistic effect is one of the strong arguments made for using variable-resistance exercises.

To decide between using isotonic or variable-resistance isotonic exercises is difficult. You have much greater freedom in deciding what muscles you will exercise in what motions you want, with isotonic. Isotonic also exercise your muscles in a more natural way by requiring balance and strength in supporting muscles. However, the most important point in strength training is not the method but the continuity of training over a long period of time. If you prefer one method over another, use it. Be confident that your pleasure at that gym with the equipment you like will give you better results than at any other facility that you do not frequent. If you do use the heavy machinery of a variable-resistance program, augment it with a good stretching routine and with strength exercises for muscles not included in the array of machines (for example, ankle flexors and trapezius muscles).

Isokinetics overcome the problems of ballistics and variance of exercise resistance with angle. In isokinetics, speed of movement is controlled by a machine. You can pull with all your might or at a fraction of your strength, but the device moves at the same speed. It is instantly adapted to anyone's level of strength and it compensates for variance in strength throughout the range of motion. It also eliminates the ballistic problem. You cannot accelerate the movement of the device. Isokinetics provide accommodating resistance that allows the exerciser to get a maximum workout at all angles of a repetition.

Few well-conducted tests have been made that compare results from isokinetic programs with those of either isotonics or isometric programs. People who have used isokinetics believe that it is possible to get a better workout and faster strength gains with isokinetics. This has not been reported in the research literature.

Isokinetics are being used in the evaluation and rehabilitation of injuries. Some professional football teams, which had been using variable-resistance isotonic equipment almost exclusively, now use isokinetic equipment, especially for players with knee injuries. Isokinetics are also being advocated for swimmers since swimming itself is an isokinetic exercise.

There is no concrete data to support the assertions that one method of training is always better than the other. It will probably be found that the three methods should be used in different situations, for different sports or even for different muscle groups. Today, however, isotonics are the most popular by far, and isotonic equipment is much more accessible to the majority of people. Therefore, when discussing specific exercises, I will mention only isotonic exercises. However, you can easily substitute isokinetic or variable-resistance isotonic exercises for most of the isotonic exercises I suggest.

EXERCISE MECHANICS

Grips

There are several grips, or methods to grasp equipment that are used in strength training. However, only two are commonly used. The first is an overhand, or pronated grip, and the second is an underhand, or supinated grip. The reason for using different grips

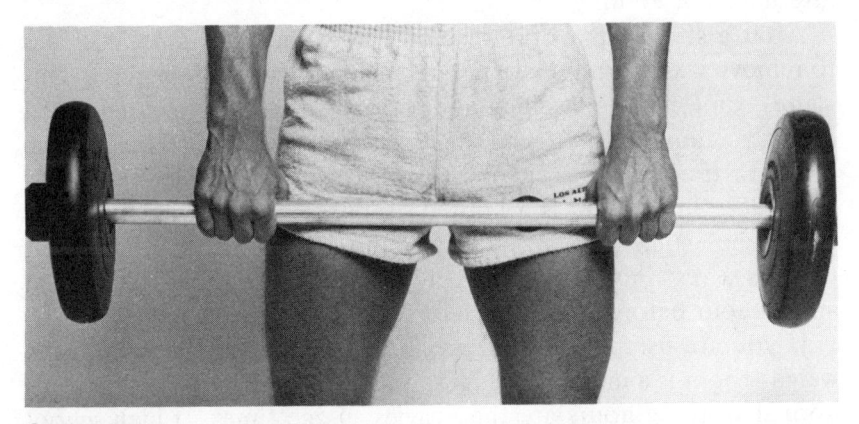

Overhand grip.

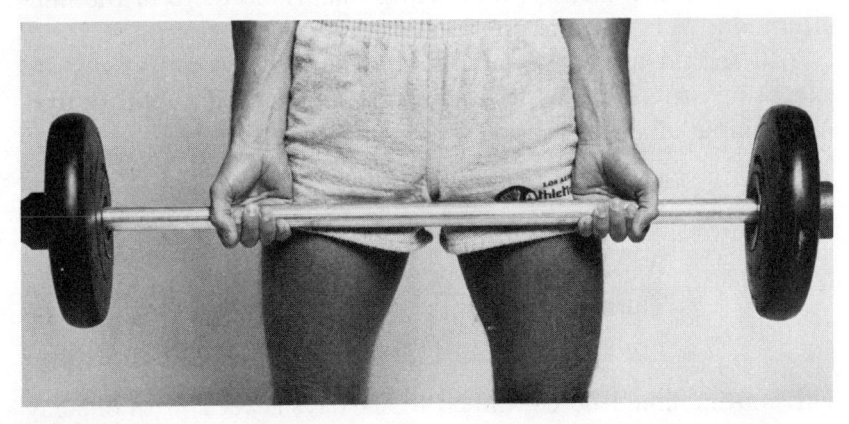

Underhand grip.

is to exercise different sets of muscles while doing nearly the same exercise. For example, while doing wrist curls with one grip only, muscles on one side of your forearm get exercise, but when the grip is reversed, muscles on the other side get a workout.

Breathing

Breathing while exercising should be at a natural cadence and cycle. Usually you will want to *exhale* while contracting muscles and *inhale* while relaxing them. The most important point is that you must not hold your breath while exerting strength.

When to work out

It is most important to schedule your workout so that you can train consistently. Picking the physiologically best-suited time of day for your workout is of no value unless you can regularly train then. If you do have freedom in scheduling workouts, try for late afternoons or evenings.

After a strenuous workout, blood flows into the muscle tissues to remove waste products generated there during the exercise. This causes some muscle swelling and, in people who have not trained recently, muscle soreness. The digestive system also needs the blood to transport the elements that were absorbed by the digestive tract. Since there is a limited supply of blood, both functions cannot be efficiently carried out at the same time. Make sure that there is a rest interval of at least an hour and a half after a meal and an hour before a meal or before going to bed.

If you are using weights or weight equipment, congestion in the weight room is a major consideration. Noon and immediately after normal working hours are the heaviest usage times. If high school students use the facility, they will probably be there in the mid-afternoon. Weight rooms are usually empty in the mornings.

You should not work out on consecutive days unless you are exercising different muscles each day. This is called a split routine. An example of a split routine is:

Monday	upper-body exercises
Tuesday	lower-body exercises
Wednesday	no workout
Thursday	upper-body exercises
Friday	lower-body exercises

This routine could be continued to six days a week, with one day for rest. This would be very strenuous and is recommended only for weight lifters with several years experience.

Three workouts a week seems to be an optimum number (unless you are doing split routines). For a maintenance program, however, even one workout a week is sufficient. At this frequency no strength gains will occur, but neither will there be significant strength losses.

Strength training should be stopped at least two days before competition. This period will allow the muscles to rest and to store glycogen, the complex sugars used as energy sources for the muscles. In preparation for long endurance events taper your strength-training program at least ten days before an event.

EXERCISE FORM

Walk into almost any weight room and you will see exercises being performed improperly. There is potential for injury in doing exercises incorrectly. More likely, however, the person exercising is not getting an efficient workout and improvements in strength will occur slowly, if at all.

The three tests of exercise form are isolation, ballistics and movement through the full range. For a muscle to be progressively overloaded, it must be isolated so that it is not being assisted by other muscles. To ensure that a muscle is isolated, watch for extraneous movements. The usual case is a large muscle group assisting a smaller, weaker group. For example, back or leg muscles may be used to accelerate a weight during an arm exercise. One of the functions of mirrors in training facilities is to enable you to watch yourself so you can eliminate extra movements.

In general, exercises should be performed through the full range of comfortable motion. Doing this helps preserve flexibility and develops strength at all points of the exercise.

Ballistics refers to exercise acceleration in the early movement of an exercise. If you accelerate very quickly, your muscles will do little or no work throughout the rest of the exercise. This practice develops strength only at the initial angle. Each repetition should be slow enough so that at each point in the movement the muscles are working to overcome the full resistance. Exceptions to this rule are made for speed training or in trying to duplicate a sports motion that may be ballistic.

The best way to ensure good exercise form is to have a friend assist you. He can rest from his workout while watching you exercise. Your partner will be able to see mistakes or sloppy movements that you may not notice. As you tire during a workout you pay less attention to form. However, no matter how tired you are, your partner gladly will tell you when you are not doing exercises correctly. His attentive stare will also dissuade you from easing off during your workout.

CHOOSING EXERCISE RESISTANCES (WEIGHTS)

Any approach to selecting the weights you use must be subjective. Your partner will probably be using different weights from you and also change his weights at different intervals. He may be using larger weights than you do in one exercise and you may use larger weights than he does in another. Choosing weights should be based solely on the individual's needs.

In general, the correct choice for a weight is that weight with which you can just achieve the desired number of repetitions. The actual poundage is of no consequence and should be of little concern in strength training. If you reach the upper limit of your repetition schedule, add weight. If you dip below the lower end of your repetition schedule, remove some weight. The key is to do the number of repetitions that your program calls for.

When starting a strength-training program choose very light weights. The most common fault for beginners is to jump into a program with too heavy a weight. Before you build strength you must know how to do the exercises. If you develop good form at first, you will probably maintain that form throughout your exercise career. After several sessions you can adjust the weights upward. Do it slowly. After several weeks of training you should be using weights that allow you to comfortably meet your program goals for repetitions.

There are several elaborate techniques for determining if you are using the correct weights. One of these uses graphs. Do several sets of the exercises, each time using different weights. Rest between sets of the same exercise. Record the weights used and the number of repetitions that you were able to perform. Then plot the work done at each exercise session on the vertical axis and the weights used on the horizontal axis. To compute the work done multiply the weight for each exercise by the number of repetitions accomplished. Assume that the distance you moved the weight was constant for each set—thus, there is no need to multiply by the distance. Drawing a line from one plotted point to the next, you should get a curve similar to the one drawn on page 15 in Chapter 2.

The highest point on the curve represents the maximum work you can do on that exercise. The area to the left of the maximum point is in the underload zone. At these weights your muscles are not being taxed enough. To the right of the maximum point, toward heavier weights, is the overload zone. Using weights in the overload zone ensures that you will develop strength efficiently. Training in the underload zone, even for long periods of time, will not result in significant gains in strength. Pick weights just to the right of or heavier than the weight under the maximum work load.

It is estimated that no strength gains will occur unless the exercise resistance is at least one-third of the maximum contraction strength. Thus, you should ensure that your weights are no less than one-third of your maximal effort for each exercise. To determine your maximum muscular strength, find the largest weight that you can lift once. This is referred to as your 1 RM (repetition maximum). Be careful when trying to find your 1 RM. Do not try this until you have learned good form on the exercise.

Often, in weight training you will find that you are not making any progress. It will seem that you are stuck with your present exercise resistances. These plateaus can be difficult to break through. Plateaus can be caused by overtraining, poor diet or lack of adequate rest. If it is not obvious that any of these is the cause, do an extra set of exercises during your next workout. An improvement in strength then suggests that you have been undertraining. If you suspect overtraining, reduce the resistance and slowly build up again.

One way to break through a plateau is to reduce the exercise resistance and increase the number of repetitions. Use the lighter weights for a minimum of three weeks and probably no longer than six weeks. Then increase the weights slowly. In a few training sessions you may be able to use heavier weights than before. You will have begun again to make progress.

WORKOUT ROUTINE

Establish a daily routine for your strength workouts. First warm up and stretch. I recommend doing a five-minute routine of stretches; then go to each exercise station and do the movements with either no weight or very little weight. Do several repetitions and move quickly onto the next exercise.

When you start your actual workout, arrange it so that you exercise the larger muscles first. The order of exercise should be legs, hips, back and stomach, chest, shoulder, upper arms, forearms, ankles and neck. While it is not essential to follow this order, it is helpful.

At each station do the first one or two repetitions with load, slowly. A large proportion of all injuries occurring in the weight room occur on the first repetition of an exercise.

When you are finished with your workout, stretch again to reduce muscle tightness.

DIET

There is so much written about diets for athletes or for people in fitness programs that I cannot begin to review the subject here. I will make only a few suggestions—ones you have undoubtedly heard before.

Eat a variety of foods from all the food groups to ensure that you are getting all the essential dietary elements. Keep fats at a low percentage of your overall caloric intake. I recommend eating 0.4 grams of protein per pound of your body weight every day. This figure is almost twice as much as the U.S. Academy of Sciences recommended in 1974 for the minimum allowance. However, active people need more protein than the minimum and it's nice to err on the excessive side rather than developing a protein deficiency. If your total caloric intake is much higher than 3000 kilocalories per day, then you need to increase your protein correspondingly.

MOTIVATION

In any training program, motivation is the key element. To develop strength, muscles must be overloaded and worked to their limit. This requires a high level of motivation at every workout. (I am not advocating all-out efforts at every workout. If you are sore or tired or maybe catching a cold, do an easy workout or even skip it. You are always the best judge of how hard to push yourself. But when you do feel good, make the most of your workout by putting forth your best effort).

It is hard to maintain the dedication to training. Too soon the promises of regular workouts are lost to early-morning blues and overcrowded schedules. Even if you can get to the training facility, your motivation may be low. It is easy to lose impetus.

The best way to combat the eventual decline in motivation is to organize or join a small group of people with similar training goals. It is then more difficult to skip a workout since you know your friends are waiting for you. Instead of going to a workout, an activity which has low priority to those not concerned with fitness, you are going to a regular appointment. Once there, everyone makes an effort to help one another. Exercise form is carefully inspected. Repetitions are counted and encouragements are given at the critical times, especially near the end of a workout when you are tired. It is at this point that you must work your hardest since the last set provides you with the greatest gains in strength, power and endurance.

The social atmosphere will quickly become the attractive force instead of the training. The goal continues to be building strength, but the formation of a group helps you toward this goal.

When contemplating a program to improve strength, many people rush out to buy a set of weights for home: "Work out in the privacy of your own home." Our experience is that the weights are used religiously—for a week or so. Then they serve merely as conversation pieces, grandiose paperweights and additional objects to be moved on cleaning day. It is the rare person who has the self-discipline to use exercise equipment regularly at home. There are just too many distractions and temptations.

If you are not sure how resolutely you will work out at home, I suggest you try an experiment before purchasing any equipment. Design a training program that requires only the facilities already available at home. Do pushups, situps, and pullups on a tree. Include about ten exercises. Try following your program for a month. If you religiously stick to it, you are one of the few who should consider buying a set of weights.

If you are like most of us, you will fail miserably. Don't waste your money on home equipment. Go to a gym where much better equipment is available. And better yet, get several friends to join you.

EXERCISE PROGRAMS

There are many exercise programs. Unfortunately, very few have been compared either with each other or with any standard. Thus the choice of programs is largely a personal one. Find one or two that suit your needs and that you enjoy doing.

The words "repetitions" and "set" have been casually used in the preceding sections of this book. But it is important to differentiate between them. A repetition is one continuous execution of an exercise. You start at a position, go through the full range of motion, and end up at the starting point. This is one repetition; one "rep" for short. A series of reps without stopping is a set. You may do five pushups and after resting a few minutes, do five more. That is described as two sets of five reps. The following exercise programs will be described in terms of reps and sets.

The number of repetitions to use in your program depends on the goals of the program. When starting an exercise program, try to do 8 - 12 repetitions. Exercise resistances should be low enough so that this number of reps can be easily accomplished. After several workouts, change the number of repetitions and the weights to match your program.

There are many suggested systems specifying the numbers of reps and sets. Professor Pat O'Shea of Oregon State University recommends the following:

Goals	Number of repetitions	Number of sets
maximum strength	1 - 3	6 - 8
strength plus	4 - 10	4 - 5
muscular endurance	12 - 20	3 - 4

As in any strength program, the weights or exercise resistance should be chosen so that the number of repetitions specified in your program can be done when you are working hard.

Other programs recommend 3 - 6 reps for strength and as many as 50 for endurance. Each coach has his or her own philosophy that will probably dictate your program. O'Shea's program appears to be reasonable and is probably a good starting point. From there you should experiment to see what gives you the best results. In general, we advocate not doing more than 20 repetitions and, actually, 12 - 15 are probably sufficient for endurance. Any more reps would guarantee that you are not in the overload zone.

John Jesse recommends a slightly different program:

Goals	Number of repetitions	Number of sets	Pace
strength	3 - 6	3 sets of 6 reps 5 sets of 5 reps 7 sets of 3 or 4 reps	slow
muscular growth	10	3 sets	slow

CHART CONTD. NEXT PAGE.

CHART CONTD. FROM PREVIOUS PAGE.

Goals	Number of repetitions	Number of sets	Pace
muscular endurance	25 - 50	1 or 2	medium
speed development	8 - 15	1 or 2	fast
power development	8 - 15	1 or 2	medium/fast

Current thinking seems to be that endurance programs build strength as well as endurance, and strength programs also build endurance. However, only a few experiments have been conducted and the established procedures of low reps for strength and higher reps for endurance are still popular.

De Lorme and Watkins believe that the following program leads to the fastest gains in strength:

Set Number	Number of repetitions	Resistance
1	10	½ 10 RM
2	10	¾ 10 RM
3	10	10 RM

Ten RM, repetition maximum, is the heaviest weight that should be used to get just 10 repetitions. One-half 10 RM is one-half of that weight. This program is thought to cause maximum hypertrophy, or muscle growth. Other researchers have suggested reducing the number of reps and increasing the exercise resistance.

Obviously we are not trying to present hard- and fast-rules for strength training. None exist, except for the principles listed in Chapter 2. Since no single program or no single combination of reps and sets can be guaranteed to produce optimal results, you must experiment during exercise and choose which program best suits your needs based on perceived results.

Here are several exercise methodologies. Again, no one is better than the other. They all have been used successfully.

PROGRESSIVE SETS

This system is well-suited for someone (especially someone who is not in good condition) who is starting a program. There are two ways to progress: increase the number of sets or increase the number of repetitions. You could start out doing one set of exercises at each workout for two to three weeks, then add a second set and continue on that schedule for the same length of time before adding the third and last set. Do not be concerned with adding weights until you have been doing three full sets for several workouts. This program minimizes muscle soreness and the possibility of injuries and allows you to work on exercise form before being concerned with strength development.

Another alternative, double progression, is to do three sets of exercises from the start but keep the number of repetitions low. Again, do not worry about the weights being used until you can do the desired number of reps throughout all three sets. Start with 8 reps for arm and shoulder exercises and 12 for legs, back and stomach.

Start with the minimum weight. Every other workout add one repetition to each set of arms and shoulder exercises and two reps to the other exercises. When you have reached a maximum of 12 reps for arms and shoulders and 20 for legs, back and stomach, increase the exercise difficulty.

In this system you perform all sets of a given exercise before going on to the next exercise. You must ensure adequate rest, at least 2 - 3 minutes, between sets. Thus, you may do all three sets of pushups before doing any pullups.

CIRCUIT TRAINING

Here we refer to circuit training not in the context of aerobic strength training (see Chapter 4), but as doing one set of each exercise in your program before doing the next set. This allows you to do your workout faster since you do not need to rest as long between successive sets. When no rest time is allowed, an aerobic workout can be achieved while strength also is developed.

PYRAMID SYSTEM

Start with an exercise resistance that is fairly light compared to your strength. Shoot for 8 - 10 repetitions during the first set. For the next set add 5 or 10 pounds so that the maximum number of repetitions you can do is lower. Continue this program three or four times until you reach the point where only two reps are possible. This is an advanced technique, one that should be attempted only if a good base of strength is possessed.

SUPER SETS

Super sets is a highly advanced technique, advocated only for those who are interested in hypertrophy. The concept here is to do a set of exercises for a particular muscle group and then, with no rest, do a set for the antagonistic muscle group. You could do bench presses closely followed by arm curls. After exercising the antagonistic pair, rest for two or three minutes, then repeat the procedure twice more. A program for super sets might consist of exercising the following pairs of antagonists.

    biceps (curls)   triceps (press)
    quadriceps (leg press)   hamstring (curls)
    chest (flies)   upper back (reverse flies)

PYRAMIDING SUPER SETS

This is an example of combining two programs. Do super sets, but after each set increase the weights.

STARTING YOUR OWN PROGRAM

If you have not used weights before and are not in good shape, start by using the simple progressive set system. Pick six to eight exercises and use weights light enough so you have no trouble in completing 8 - 12 repetitions. Do only one set for the first two weeks. Then add a second set and eventually a third.

By this time you will feel comfortable doing the exercises. Increase the exercise resistance slowly so that you can do only 3 - 6 repetitions in each of the three sets. Stay on this schedule for at least six weeks. If you desire, add exercises to make a total of 10.

You can develop strength, power or endurance one at a time. After you have a good base of strength, you can work on power or endurance, as you wish. But continue on one program for a minimum of six weeks. Do the exercises in circuit-training sets. Use the more advanced systems only after months of experience.

Here are my recommendations for reps and sets.

Goals	Number of repetitions	Number of sets	Pace
learning exercises	8 - 12	1 - 3	slow
strength	3 - 6	3 - 4	slow
endurance	15 - 20	3	medium
general fitness	8 - 12	3	medium

To develop muscular power—the rapid application of strength—do the exercises at a fast pace. Try to explode the weight upward, even when the muscle is tired and cannot contract quickly.

4

Aerobic Strength Training

Circuit training is ...."utilized mainly for the development of all-around muscular and circulo-respiratory efficiency. It appears to be best suited for the development of a general state of fitness."

—Sorani

Many strength-training programs are geared to improving muscular strength of a few motions needed in a sport, but cardiovascular development does not occur since repetitions are performed slowly and a rest period is taken between each set. Aerobic strength training, or circuit training, develops strength and cardiovascular fitness at the same time.

The element of time is instrumental in transforming an anaerobic strength-training program into an aerobic one. A vigorous exercise pace is continued for a long time period (longer than 10 minutes), thus ensuring aerobic conditioning. For cardiovascular training effects, that is, for improvement in conditioning to occur, the heart rate must be elevated beyond a threshold value. Experiments have shown this threshold value to be equal to a person's resting pulse rate plus 60 percent of the difference between their maximum and their resting pulse rate. (The maximum heart rate is defined later.) Although this value may be achieved or even exceeded in conventional strength training, the heart rate falls below the value between sets. For aerobic training to occur, the heart rate must exceed the threshold for an extended period of time and thus most strength-training programs are anaerobic.

Aerobic training can be achieved by using time in one of two ways. A goal can be to do a fixed number of repetitions at each exercise and try to minimize the total time required to finish the workout. This is the concept used in outdoor circuit-training courses, also called parcourses and fitness trails. This method lends itself well to using fixed stations and running from one station to the next. It is not recommended in a weight room, where an overzealous attempt to minimize elapsed time could result in an injury.

Most outdoor circuit-training courses (OCTC) are geared toward serving the general public in fitness programs. A disadvantage is that the selection of exercises cannot be changed and the degree of difficulty for most of the exercises cannot be changed. Thus, progressive resistance—gradually increasing exercise resistance as a person gets stronger—cannot be implemented. However, OCTC's are useful for the athlete in training, as well as for the person interested in fitness, for a change of pace in training or as part of a strength maintenance program. Running an OCTC on a sunny spring day is a great reward after training indoors throughout the winter. Also, if you stop strength training either during the competitive season or in the offseason, use of an OCTC on a weekly basis will help maintain your strength at a high level.

For weight-room workouts the second method of timing is preferred. Instead of trying to minimize the total time taken to do a fixed number of repetitions, you should try to maximize the number of repetitions in a fixed time period. This requires a timer to tell you when to start and stop each exercise.

There are several benefits to aerobic strength training in addition to developing strength and aerobic conditioning simultaneously. Aerobic programs are so adaptable that they can be used by almost anyone. Only those who are in poor physical condition should not use these techniques. Weights or exercise difficulty (for example, the height of a situp board) can be varied to match anyone's level of strength. The intensity of the workout, that is, the aspect of movement, can be varied to match a person's cardiovascular condition. The exercise duration of each set can be varied, the number of exercises can be increased or decreased and the number of sets of exercises can be changed.

Although usually geared to give a general workout, aerobic strength-training programs, especially weight-room circuit training,

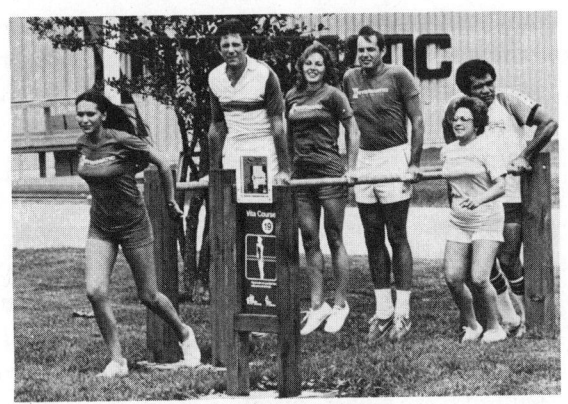

Parcourses are outdoor circuit training.

can be modified to fit the specific needs of a sport. The exercises used in the workout can be matched to the strength requirements of a sport and the exercise duration also can be varied to more closely match that of a particular event. A sprinter might want a short exercise period with fewer repetitions at higher weights. The middle-distance runner might opt for an exercise duration closer to the duration of his event, using lighter weights and more repetitions.

An advantage of aerobic strength training is that a group of people can train at the same time with less confusion than occurs with a disorganized mob in the weight room. The high intensity of the structured workouts allows a large number of people to train quickly. From a weight-room manager's point of view it provides an efficient and maximum utilization of the facilities. From the participant's point of view it gives a vigorous workout in a short time.

A group of up to 25 people can easily work out at the same time, even in a small facility. Usually each person will do the same exercises, but individual preferences can be accommodated, provided that they do not interfere with the other participants. The key is to have everyone know what the workout plan is and to assist one another in changing weights and setting equipment. Weight machines are conducive to this style of training in that weights can be changed in an instant and there is little danger of injury due to weights falling off barbells.

No system is perfect, and to get the benefits of aerobic strength training you must give up something. Although this program develops both strength and cardiovascular conditioning, it probably does not develop them as fast as could individual, traditional training programs. With aerobic strength programs, as you push toward your cardiovascular limits you will not be able to push to your muscular limits. Thus, strength development will occur less rapidly and ultimate strength gains may be limited by your cardiovascular endurance. Also, although aerobic conditioning occurs, the duration of workout (15 - 30 minutes) may not be long enough for people interested in developing the very long endurance found in distance swimmers or marathon runners.

Thus, aerobic strength programs are a compromise between strength development and cardiovascular development. However, it may be the optimum compromise and is an excellent method for achieving a high level of general fitness. When complimented by LSD-type (long, slow distance) exercise—running, swimming, cycling or cross-country skiing—or by a combination of such exercises along with a stretching routine, a very high level of all-around fitness can be achieved.

One more asset of aerobic strength training is its popularity. People enjoy the feeling of having a strenuous workout; they appreciate the short time the workout takes; and they develop comradeship with others who are working out. At the Boulder YMCA, in Colorado, we have as many participants in aerobic strength training as we can handle. No matter what time of day we hold classes (6:30 a.m. to 9:00 p.m.) passersby stop to watch and rarely does a week go by without one or more of the observers asking to join us.

INDOOR CIRCUIT TRAINING*

Aerobic strength training, with a fixed exercise time, requires either someone timing the participants or time being announced by a timing system (a cassette recorder with a timed tape does a good job). The people working out exert their maximum effort during the exercise time and then, without resting, move to the next exercise. There are usually between 8 and 16 exercises in a

---

* I am using the terms "indoor" and "outdoor" to describe the two systems of circuit training. The difference between the two methods is really one of timing, not location.

circuit, or set, and each circuit is usually done three times. It is an exhausting exercise routine, but one that is especially enjoyed by athletes who participate in endurance sports.

Any isotonic or isokinetic exercise can be incorporated into this aerobic system. Use the same exercises that you would use in conventional weight training. When first starting an aerobic weight training program choose a small number of exercises, eight for example. After several weeks you can gradually increase the number of exercises. Do not include more than two exercises for similar muscle groups, and keep apart exercises that work the same muscle groups. If you perform each set of exercises correctly, the muscle group will be near or at muscle fatigue, and doing a similar exercise before the muscle can recover will accomplish nothing.

The exercises used in this or any other weight-training program need not always be the same. Changing the routine can make the workout more interesting. You might use cardiovascular exercises in your circuit in addition to strength exercises. For example, you could run, do jumping jacks, or pedal a stationary bicycle for a minute or longer between circuits.

The order in which you do the exercises is largely dependent on the layout of the facility you use. Since the amount of time allowed between exercises is short, an exercise station should be close to the preceding station. Also, if several people are working out together, exercises should be arranged to minimize traffic flow problems. If possible, lay out the exercises so everyone is always moving in the same direction—either clockwise or counterclockwise. Because this is a very strenuous and exhausting program, people often forget where to go next; the simpler the system, the better.

If a large facility is available to you, you can spread the exercises out to have people move briskly from one station to the next. This requires good workout coordination and assistance in getting equipment ready. It is recommended more as a change of pace than for a regular workout.

Even if you use weight machines, assistance in setting weights and equipment is desirable and sometimes necessary. People working out can help each other, but additional assistance makes the workout more efficient. One way to do this is to break up a group into two—one sets weights while the other exercises.

Choosing the time base to use is the most important element in planning aerobic training. I recommend using a base of 30 seconds—that is, each exercise will be started on the half-minute. Exercis are performed for 10, 15 or 20 seconds depending on the current conditioning of each individual. The remaining part of the 30 seconds is used to move to the next exercise and get in position.

The half-minute time base seems to be ideal for general conditioning. Using 20 seconds for exercising (and 10 seconds for moving to the next station) allows you enough time to get in an optimum number of repetitions, 8 - 15, before muscle fatigue. Longer exercise time would be wasted unless you decreased your weights and did more repetitions. In this case you would no longer be exercising in the optimum repetition range and strength gains would come more slowly.

Another factor to consider is your heart rate. Aerobic strength training is designed to elevate your heart rate and to keep it elevated over a long (longer than 10 minutes) time period. Long time bases may allow your heart to drop below optimum cardiovascular training levels (see below).

Deviate from the half-minute time base if you want to match your exercise duration to that of the sport you are training for. For example, a 100-meter sprinter may want to train for 10 - 12 seconds. A tennis player may want to exercise for 15 or 30 seconds. Experiment with different time bases and compare how you feel and how you do in competition.

It is interesting to monitor your heart rate after exercising and at other times of the day. A healthy heart is one that can respond quickly to the demands placed on it. When the demands are reduced, it should be able to return quickly to near its normal rate. Take your pulse immediately after exercising. You can continue to count your pulse every minute or so after finishing to see how quickly it returns. It should drop to below 100 beats per minute (from a high of around 140) within three minutes of finishing exercising. Also, it should drop to within five beats per minute of your pre-exercise pulse, in half an hour.

To gain cardiovascular benefit the heart rate should be elevated beyond your critical training level. On the other hand, if the pulse rate is too high, physical injury could occur. One estimate of a person's threshold value is the sum of his resting pulse plus 60 percent of the difference between this pulse and his maximum pulse. A less accurate measure, but one that is more commonly used, is 70 - 80 percent of the maximum heart rate. The upper limit for optimum cardiovascular training is 85 percent of the maximum heart rate.

A person's maximum heart rate can be estimated by a cardiologist from the results of a stress EKG test. Without having done this test, an estimate can be made as follows:

Maximum heart rate = 220 - (your age)

For example, if you are 30 years old your maximum heart rate is estimated to be 190 beats per minute. Your cardiovascular threshold value would be 138 provided that your resting pulse was 60 beats per minute. The optimum range for aerobic conditioning would be about 133 - 152 beats a minute. Note that there is a slight difference between the extimates calulated from these two rules of thumb.

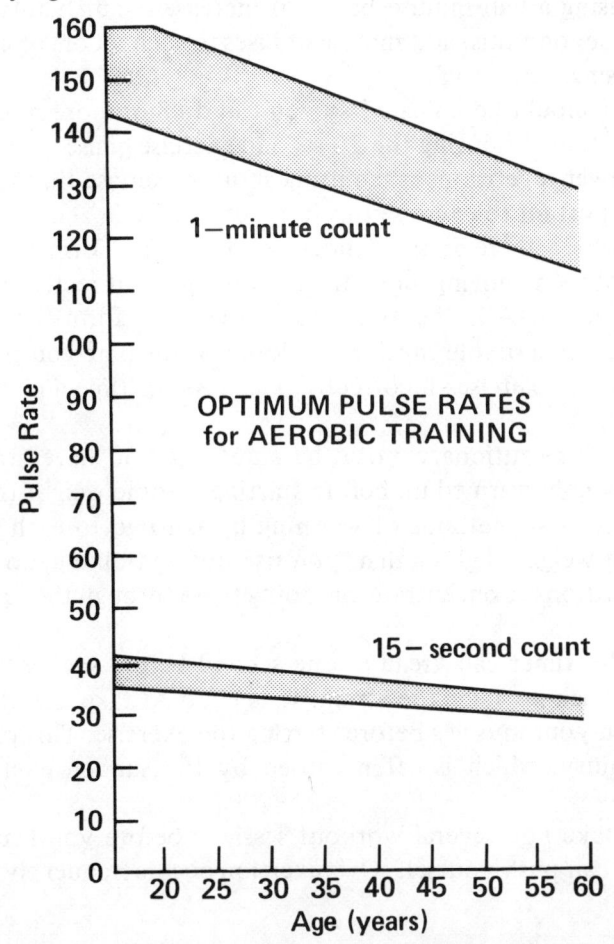

Optimum pulse rates for aerobic training are shown in the accompanying chart. Pulse rates are shown both for a minute count and a 15-second count. Because your pulse rate will drop quickly when you stop exercising, use a 15-second count to estimate your exercise pulse rate.

If you take a pulse count after any strenuous activity (for example, after running a race) you will develop a feel for your optimum exercise heart range. Abnormal pulse counts should be discussed with your physician.

Using the half-minute time base, you should actively exercise for between 10 and 20 seconds. Starting out, you should use the 10-second period until you feel comfortable exercising through 3 full sets. Gradually increase the time you exercise (therby decreasing the time available for getting to the next station). Add 5-second increments of exercise duration to the third set, a few exercises at a time. Then gradually increase the exercise time in the preceding sets. The maximum advisable exercise time is 20 seconds using a half-minute base. To increase the difficulty of the workout beyond this, add more exercises to each set or concentrate on increasing your weights.

Weights should be adjusted so you can do 8 or more repetitions but fewer than 15 during the 20-second exercise phase. You should aim for fewer repetitions when using shorter exercise times.

It is important to exercise carefully, especially in aerobic weight training where there is the tendency to sacrifice form for speed. Concentrate on moving only those body parts directly involved in the exercise. Ask the timer to watch your form—he will be able to see undesirable motion or sloppy form that you may not notice. Doing exercises incorrectly is a waste of time and can lead to injuries.

Another precautionary note: be sure that you have stretched and thoroughly warmed up before starting aerobic weight training. One of the best methods of warming up is to go to each station and, using weights lighter than you use during training, do several slow repetitions. Concentrate on doing these through the full range of motion.

Have the timer call "ready" one second before saying "go" to tell you when to take the strain. It is good to take the strain of weights on your muscles before starting the exercise. This prevents muscle injury, which is often caused by the sudden exertion of lifting.

It will take you several workout sessions before you learn how hard you can push yourself. Overexertion occurs frequently among new participants. They feel dizzy or can even get nauseous. You are advised to start slowly and gradually increase your effort. If you do feel woozy, drop out immediately—do not continue: the feeling will not go away if you keep working out.

You may want to test yourself periodically to check your progress. Since aerobic strength training is a combination of training for strength plus cardiovascular conditioning, you may want to test each component separately. Timing yourself for a mile-and-a-half run (Cooper's test) can suffice to show improvements in your aerobic conditioning. For measuring gains in strength, do a two-minute exercise test on the bench press, situps and leg press. Do as many repetitions as you can in this time, using exercise resistances lower than those you use during training. Make sure that you record the exercise resistance so that you can compare your results over a period of time.

The easiest way to test for strength gains is to record the number of repetitions that you can do for each exercise during a workout. Keeping a record of your results also will allow you to see the impact on your training from other factors (for example, loss of sleep or overtraining). When comparing numbers of repetitions performed with different weights, multiply the weight used by the number of repetitions. This gives values of the work performed that can be compared when using different exercise resistances.

OUTDOOR CIRCUIT TRAINING

An outdoor circuit-training course (OCTC) is a set of exercise stations along a running path. The stations are usually separated by at least 100 yards but by not more than 300 yards. People

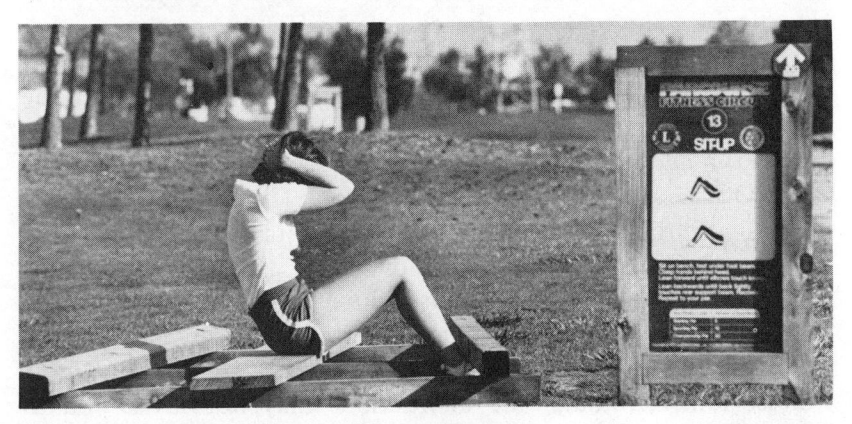

Parcourses are found on many college campuses.

using the course run from one station to the next, and do a specified number of repetitions at each station.

This type of aerobic strength training is often called parcours or fitness trail training. Over the last decade it has gone from near obscurity to fast-growing popularity. Its rise in adherents parallels the running boom. People out for a jog can get in some strength training by running through a parcourse.

Although most often found outside, aerobic/strength courses can be used indoors. Chinning, pushups, horse vaulting or other stations can be laid out around the perimeter of a gymnasium.

Usually a person selects as at each station one of three levels of intensity for a workout. The number of repetitions that correspond to that level of intensity are specified. You are told to start out on the lowest level (fewest repetitions) and work up to the highest level. At the same time, you try to reduce the total time required to run the course.

A range of exercise difficulty is built into many of the stations. For example, a pushup station can be built at three or more levels. The tallest bar makes pushups relatively easy; at the shorter bars, pushups are more difficult. (Although this variability is possible, many commercially produced OCTC's do not have it.) Thus, the difficulty of the exercise and the number of repetitions can be varied while still trying to minimize the total elapsed time.

Most outdoor circuits are laid along a mile to a mile-and-a-half of running path and consist of 12 - 20 exercise stations. They usually take 12 - 20 minutes to run. Thus, workouts are intense but are of short duration. To orient workouts toward longer endurance training, a course can be run more than once. To do this the participant will want to lower the exercise difficulty or the number of repetitions from the levels normally used. One scheme for doing an extended workout is to run the course three times, but on the second circuit run the course without doing the exercises. The middle run allows time for some muscle recovery.

An OCTC can be used for competition. The total time needed to finish a circuit is a good measure of a person's overall fitness—that is, their strength and cardiovascular fitness. Competition should be attempted only by those who are in good physical shape and who have run the exercise trail and know how demanding it is.

Instructions are provided on posted signs at the start of most fitness trails. Although the instructions may not advise you to stretch before starting, you certainly should. A short jog or set of bounding or skipping exercises is also recommended before starting. Once on the course, move at a comfortable pace. You will find that the exercises raise your heart rate and the run between stations will allow it to return to a sustainable, aerobic rate.

Most courses are designed to give you a gradual buildup in intensity, which tapers off near the end.

Exercise course materials can be purchased from one of several companies; however, you might want to save money and build your own course. Buying from the manufacturers is quite expensive.

The biggest expense for OCTC's is the instructional signs. In fact, if you study commercially constructed equipment you will see most manufacturers produce elaborate signs and much less elaborate equipment. Signs need not be fancy. Hand-painted or wood-routed signs are relatively cheap and do the job.

Also, when you buy from manufacturers, most will ship the equipment from a warehouse and you will have no choice in the selection of exercises, the number of exercise stations or the size of the equipment.

The most serious drawback of the commercially designed courses is that they mix stretching with strength-building exercises. Stretching should be done before and after each workout, but manufacturers insert several stretching stations along the trail. The number of stretching exercises is too few and reduces the number of stations available for strength training. Also, it is impossible to take time to stretch properly if you are trying to reduce your overall time or to compete against others. Place the stretching signs near the start and finish of your course instead, and include at least 10 exercises designed to stretch a variety of muscles. The exercises in the strength-training course should be kept solely for strength training.

USES OF AEROBIC STRENGTH TRAINING

Aerobic strength training is meant to be used as an adjunct to a general fitness program. It encourages flexibility and develops muscle strength and endurance. It has value by itself, but is best when it compliments other longer-duration endurance exercises— for example, running, swimming or cycling.

Aerobic strength training is also valuable for sports training in preseason or during the season. If a conventional strength training program is being used in the offseason, aerobic strength training allows the strength gained to be maintained while endurance is improved prior to the sport's season. It allows for the transfer to occur from low-repetition strength to endurance. During the competitive season, workouts once or twice a week ensure strength maintenance and don't detract from the training specific to your sport.

Strength training is good for endurance-sport athletes. Runners who may fear adding muscle mass with conventional weight training can use aerobic strength training instead. Any increase in muscle mass will be slight and will probably not impair running performance. However, the increase in strength can help performance.

5

Strength Exercises

In this chapter we present exercises for strength training. Weights or weight machines are recommended for most of the exercises. This is because equipment allows you to isolate an exercise to a particular motion and thus to a particular muscle or muscle group. By isolating, I mean that the action of the exercise is being accomplished only by the desired muscle or muscles, without assistance from other muscles. Isolation allows for an intensive workout of a particular muscle, which is necessary for overall muscle development and strength gain.

By using weights you can select the resistance appropriate for your current level of strength and gradually increase the resistance of the exercise. This is fundamentally important in progressively overloading a muscle. Also, many people cannot do even one repetition of some exercises when using their body weight for resistance. The best example is chinups. People who cannot do chinups can start developing muscle tone and strength by using light dumbbells or barbells. With time they can become strong enough to do chinups.

For these reasons strength training is often synonymous with weight training; however, there are many good strength training exercises that do not require weights. Also, there are many times when you may not have access to weights. You can substitute comparable exercises that do not use weights when on business trips or vacation. Thus, we have included both types of exercises in this chapter.

The number of exercises that can be performed using weight equipment, especially with unrestricted equipment like barbells and dumbbells, is limitless; however, there are in most cases only a few exercises that isolate a particular muscle or group. These are the ones shown here. Exercises for particular sports that do not isolate single muscle groups are described in the following chapter.

Although we have discussed the isolation of muscles as a fundamental of strength training, it is difficult to devise exercises that isolate a single muscle. Several muscles are usually engaged in any single motion and it is impractical, if not impossible, to isolate an action to one particular muscle. For example, there are four muscles in the quadriceps femoris group that all contribute to extending the lower leg. Motions of the foot are activated by over 20 muscles or muscle groups. Twenty-two muscles provide movement for the hip joint.

Two points become clear from the above numeration of muscles. Unless you are a professional, you probably do not need (or want) to know the names of all the muscles in the body. If you are interested in learning these, see the bibliography to find a book on kinesiology—the science of movement. The second point is that the isolation of individual muscles is not desirable—there are not enough hours in a day to exercise each individual muscle.

Instead of isolating individual muscles in strength training, you try to isolate individual motions. Since joints allow motion in restricted planes or directions, exercises are devised that work the muscles producing movement in these planes. If you analyze how each part of your body moves or rotates, you will learn what motions should be mimicked in strength training.

For example, motions of the lower arm relative to the upper arm are restricted by the elbow joint. You can bend (flex) your arm or straighten (extend) it. Extension is accomplished by two muscles (triceps brachii and anconeus), and flexing is accomplished by four (biceps brachii, brachioradialis, brachialis and pronator teres). In exercising these muscles, however, you need to consider only the motion, not the individual muscles. Thus, you select a minimum of two exercises — one that strengthens the extensors and one that strengthens the flexors.

For most motions there are a number of exercises that could be selected. Even for one exercise, a great deal of variation can be accomplished by changing the grip or foot stance, etc. Exercises should be adjusted either to more closely mimic the motions of a sport or just to work the muscles at a slightly different angle.

Varying the exercises also relieves the boredom of following the same routine over a long period of time.

The exercises presented in this chapter are divided into 10 exercise groups based on motions of the body. These groups are subdivided into two or more sets of exercises. The purpose of subdivision is to emphasize that each member of an opposing pair of muscles should be exercised. If you are exercising the extensors of the arm, you should exercise the flexors of the arm. As pointed out in previous chapters, balance between opposing muscles prevents injuries and promotes good posture.

The motions, which have been used to categorize the exercises, are described as follows. Flexion and extension are opposing actions. In flexion, the angle between the body parts decreases — that is, the body parts are brought closer together. Extension is the opposite motion — the angle increases between two body parts. Hyperextension is the continuing of the extension motion beyond a straight line. For example, when you bend over to touch your toes, you are flexing your trunk. Standing up is an extension of the trunk. Hyperextension would be the arching of your back.

The second pair of opposing actions is abduction and adduction. In abduction, the motion is away from the centerline of the body. Raising your foot out to the side (while keeping your leg straight) is an abduction of the hip joint. Bringing the leg back toward the centerline is adduction.

These four terms describe most of the motions; however, there are several others, like rotation. You can rotate your upper body while keeping your feet fixed, or you can rotate your wrist and lower arm.

The ankle joint is capable of motion around three axes. Bringing the toes upward is known as dorsiflexion — we will call this ankle flexion. Pushing them downward is plantar flexion — we will call this ankle extension. Inversion is the rotation of the foot up to the inside and eversion is the pulling of the foot up to the outside. The ankle joint also allows rotation; you can rotate your feet while they are flat on the floor.

These terms will be used in identifying exercises instead of using names of the muscles. Strength training is less complicated if you remember motions and not muscles. Also, if you think of movement and ensure that each movement in your exercise routine has an opposing movement represented, you will maintain a natural balance between opposing muscles.

STRENGTH TRAINING EXERCISE GROUPS

Group	Principal Muscles
1a Leg extension	Quadriceps
1b Leg flexion	Hamstring group
2a Hip extension	Gluteus maximus
2b Hip flexion	Iliacus, psoas, pectineus
3a Leg abduction	Gluteus medius, tensor fasciae latae
3b Leg adduction	Adductor magnus, longus, brevis
4a Trunk extension	Erector spinae
4b Trunk flexion	Abdominals (including obliques)
5a Arm extension	Triceps
5b Arm flexion	Biceps
6a Arm abduction	Trapezius
6b Arm adduction	Pectorals
7a Arm elevation	Deltoid
7b Arm depression	Latissiumus dorsi
7c Shoulder elevation	Upper trapezius
7d Shoulder depression	Lower trapezius
8a Ankle extension	Gastrocnemius
8b Ankle flexion	Tibialis anterior
8c Ankle eversion	Peroneus brevis and longus
8d Ankle inversion	Tibialis anterior
9a Wrist extension	Forearm extensors
9b Wrist flexion	Forearm flexors
9c Finger grip	Forearm and finger muscles
10a Neck extension	Splenius capitis, cervicis
10b Neck flexion	Scaleni muscles, Sterno-mastoid

STRENGTH TRAINING EXERCISE GROUPS

Location	Action
Front of thigh	Extends lower leg relative to upper leg
Back of thigh	Pulls the lower leg up to the rear
Buttocks	Pulls upper leg to the rear
Front of hip	Pulls upper leg forward
Outside of hip and upper leg	Pulls the leg to the outside away from the body's centerline
Inner surface of upper leg and hip, groin	Pulls legs together
Along back	Straightens the spine
Front of abdominal cavity	Flexes the spine—bends the upper body
Back of upper arm	Straightens the arm at the elbow
Front of upper arm	Flexes the arm at the elbow
Upper back	Pulls the shoulder blades together
Chest	Pulls arms together in front of chest
Top of upper arm	Raises the arm upward
Middle of back	Pulls the arms downward
Neck, top of shoulder	Pulls collarbone upward
Upper back	Pulls the collarbone down
Calf	Pulls the heel upward
Front of lower leg	Pulls foot upward
Outside of lower leg	Pulls foot to the outside
Inside of lower leg	Pulls foot to the inside
Back of forearm	Pulls wrist upward
Underside of forearm	Pulls wrist toward underside
Forearm and hand	Opens and closes the fist
Back of neck	Pulls head backward
Neck to upper ribs	Pulls head forward

54 STRENGTH EXERCISES

Common muscle names are given for most exercises; however, the listing of names is not meant to be definitive. In most cases only the superficial muscles, those lying closest to the surface, will be mentioned. See the chart and figure for the locations and action of major muscle groups.

With strengthening exercises for each muscle group we have included a set of stretching exercises. We did not attempt to give a complete stretching program but have presented a few stretches that should follow a strength workout.

There are five main benefits of a stretching program: 1) Increased flexibility — the ability to move through the full range of possible motion. 2) Prevention of injuries — stretching reduces the possibility of muscle pulls. 3) Elimination of muscle stiffness. 4) Increased body relaxation. 5) Increased muscle power — although strength is not increased by stretching, stretching allows faster muscle contraction and thus greater power.

Stretches should be performed as static exercises rather than as ballistic or bouncing exercises. The advantages of the static over

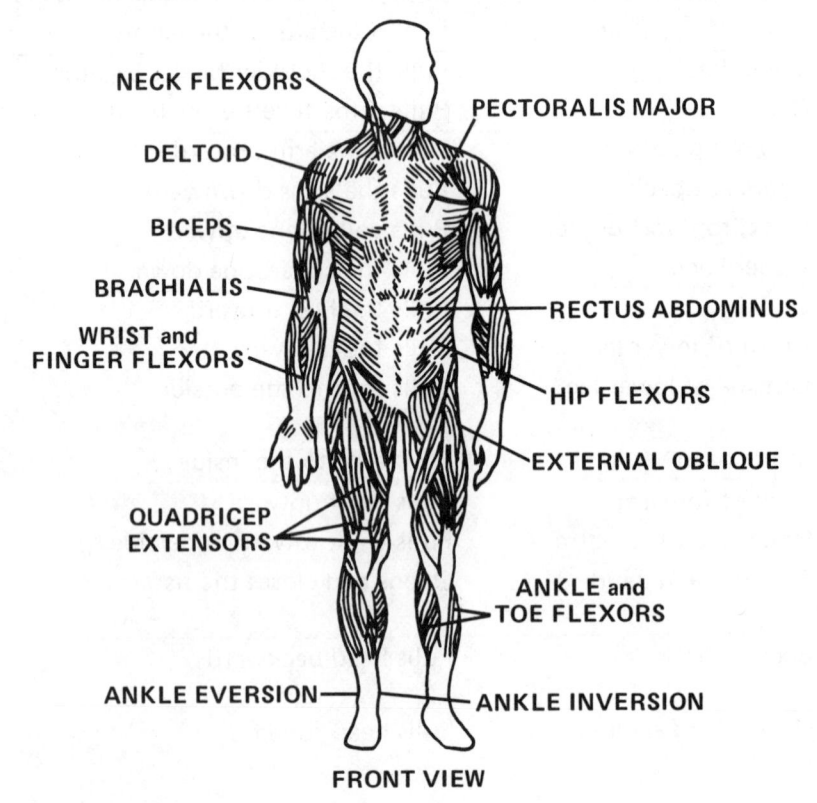

FRONT VIEW

- NECK FLEXORS
- PECTORALIS MAJOR
- DELTOID
- BICEPS
- BRACHIALIS
- WRIST and FINGER FLEXORS
- RECTUS ABDOMINUS
- HIP FLEXORS
- EXTERNAL OBLIQUE
- QUADRICEP EXTENSORS
- ANKLE and TOE FLEXORS
- ANKLE EVERSION
- ANKLE INVERSION

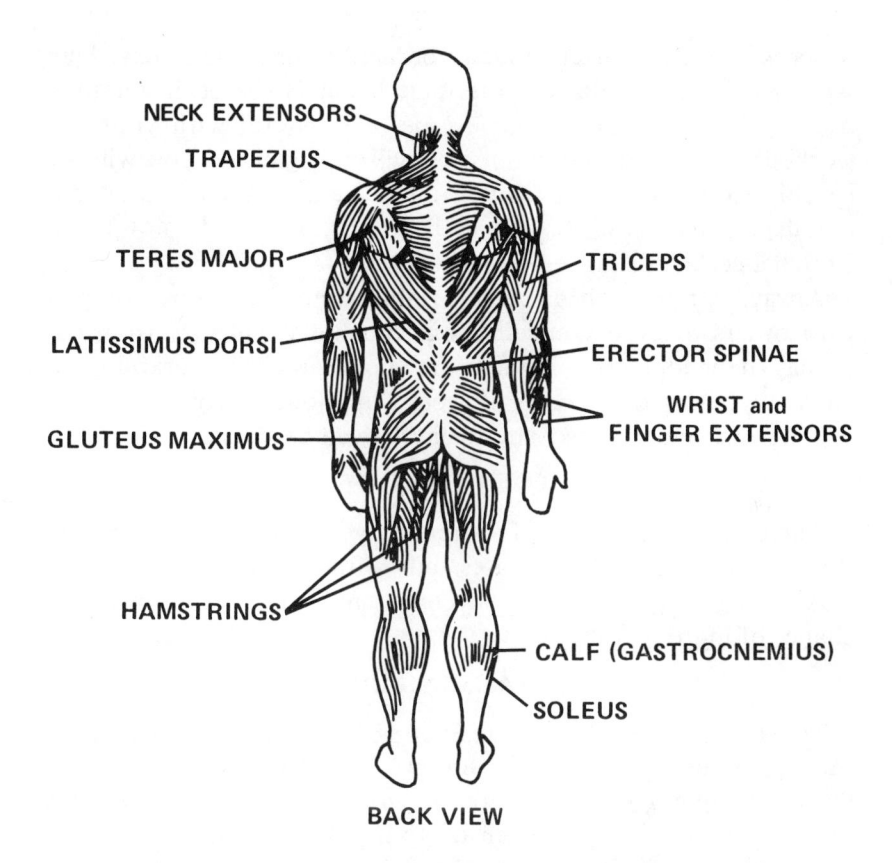

NECK EXTENSORS
TRAPEZIUS
TERES MAJOR
LATISSIMUS DORSI
GLUTEUS MAXIMUS
TRICEPS
ERECTOR SPINAE
WRIST and FINGER EXTENSORS
HAMSTRINGS
CALF (GASTROCNEMIUS)
SOLEUS

BACK VIEW

the ballistic method are: muscle injury is much more likely due to overstretching when using the ballistic method. The ballistic method tends to cause muscle soreness rather than to reduce it — the opposite of the static method.

Each stretch should be held in a comfortable position for 15 to 30 seconds. A comfortable position is one in which you feel the stretching sensation but do not feel pain. If your breathing becomes irregular, you probably have stretched too far.

While doing static stretching, the stretch sensation should dissipate. If it does not, you probably have stretched too far. Next time be a bit more conservative. If, at the end of the stretching exercise, the sensation has significantly decreased, increase the stretch slightly. Hold this new position for another 15 to 30 seconds. Then relax.

Stretching should be done before weight training to loosen the muscles and prevent injuries. It should be repeated afterward—this is your preparation for the next workout. In general it is better to work out at, or after, midday because your muscles have been stretched somewhat during your daily living. However, if you must train early in the morning, be especially careful with your pre-workout stretching. Your muscles will be tight and you will not be able to stretch as far as you might be accustomed to later in the day. Stretch only as far as is comfortable — do not try to stretch a certain distance or angle.

Always stretch within comfortable limits. Do not compete with others or even yourself. Your flexibility will vary from day to day depending on temperature, your previous workout, etc. Gradually, over the course of weeks or months, your flexibility will increase and the associated benefits will be yours.

THE WORKOUT

There are three phases of a strength workout. Too many people skip the first and third phases, but without them you will not make as rapid progress as you could, and you take an increased chance of injuring yourself.

WARMING UP

The warm-up period prepares your head, heart and muscles for the strenuous exercises that follow. By preparing your head, I mean planning a realistic workout and becoming mentally ready to exert yourself. Preparation of your voluntary and involuntary (heart) muscles is the process of making the transition from a low to a high level of activity.

If you have not planned your workout prior to arrival at the weight room, you should plan it while you warm up. You should know what exercises you are going to do, what sequence you will do them in and what resistance you will use. When first starting out in a new exercise program, it is best to write down your plan in advance. Carry your plan with you and note the repetitions you do. This gives you the information you need to modify your plan.

Also, when starting a program, or when returning to a program after several weeks or longer of layoff, start with a conservative workout. Set goals below what you think you can do and certainly do not try to regain your former strength in one workout. If your body responds well to the first two or three workouts, gradually intensify your program.

If you have not used weights before, start off with 6-8 exercises. Use very light weights so that the exercises are easy to perform. The first few sessions should be geared to learning how to do the exercises properly and not toward strength development.

It is hoped that by planning your workout in advance, you will select a realistic routine and objectives. It is important to match your performance with your goals. This way you can determine whether or not your plan is realistic. Make modifications along the way as you see fit.

After mental preparation, you must get your heart and cardiovascular system ready for the workout. If you have been sitting in an office or classroom all day, your pulse is probably slow and not ready for a heavy workout. Walk briskly to the gym and do several minutes of mild exercise (for example, jumping jacks). The idea is not to tire yourself or to work up a sweat, but to elevate your pulse.

This phase of warmup is going to raise your body temperature, and the body is able to exert more strength when its temperature is raised. There are no set time lengths for the warmup; however, one to three minutes seems to be the correct range.

The third period of the warmup is the longest. It is reserved for stretching your muscles. Prior to exercising, muscles are often tight — stretching will relieve this tightness and prepare the muscles for subsequent strength training.

I recommend one additional pre-exercise step, especially when you plan to use heavy weights. Do one set of the exercises in your program with very light weights. Do two or three slow repetitions, concentrating on your form and on achieving full extension and contraction. After this you are ready to start your strength workout.

DURING THE WORKOUT

During the workout you should concentrate on fully extending and contracting each movement, which aids in maintaining flexibility. Do the exercises slowly enough so that you are not jerking or bouncing the weights. Be especially careful in the first repetition so that you do not explode the weights upward — the first repetition is when many injuries occur, especially if there has not been a good warmup.

If you injure yourself during a workout, stop! Do not try to work it off. Very often you can prevent potentially serious damage to a muscle by stopping. Minor injuries heal quickly and may cause you to miss only one or two workouts or maybe even none. But by pushing yourself and further exercising the injury, you can cause a more serious injury, which could take much longer to heal.

In addition to muscle injuries, there is another class of injury that often occurs during a workout. The usual cause is impatience, and the victims are toes and fingers. Make sure collars are securely fastened onto barbells and dumbbells. Do not assume that the previous user left them secured. Also, do not reach your hand through weight machinery apparatus. If the machine gets hung up somehow, remove the load before trying to fix the machine.

WARMDOWN

To reduce or prevent muscle soreness, the warmdown is the most important part of the workout. You should thoroughly stretch your muscles after you train. The workout caused your muscles to become tight — stretching will loosen them.

Muscle soreness accompanies any significant increase in muscle use. It is caused by the accumulation of wastes in the muscle. As the muscle adjusts to the increased levels of work, circulation in the muscle will improve, which will speed up the elimination of wastes. If you are starting a training program, you can expect your muscles to be sore after the first few workouts. Do not be concerned with this soreness — the only effective way to eliminate it is to continue on your exercise schedule. If you skip a few sessions due to the soreness, your muscles will not adapt to the workouts and you will never overcome soreness.

To reduce soreness try stretching, heat and massage. Apply the heat for about 20 to 30 minutes at a time. Heat relaxes the muscles and increases blood circulation, which can remove waste products from the muscle.

WEIGHT EQUIPMENT

Essential for almost any strength-training program is a set of dumbbells and barbells. These may be the only equipment used in a program but more often they compliment weight machines. The beauty of dumbbells and barbells is their versatility and low cost.

Dumbbells are held one in each hand. Fixed-weight dumbbells come in five-pound increments. With variable-weight dumbbells you add weights just like you do with a barbell.

Barbells consist of a steel bar, a spacing sleeve, inside and outside locking collars, and weights. When using barbells, ensure that the collars are securely fastened so that the weights will not slide off.

Weight machines are much more complicated. There are about a dozen major manufacturers of weight machines and they all make

One dumbbell for each hand.

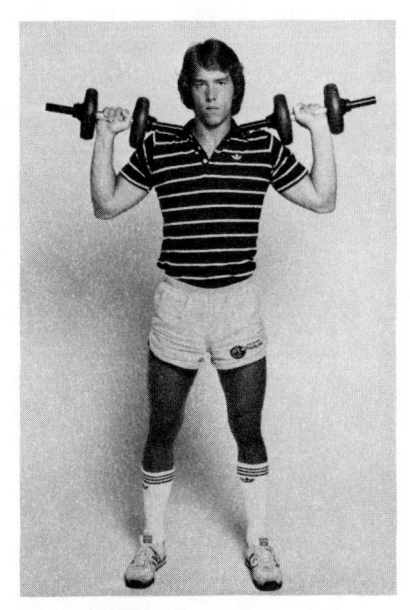

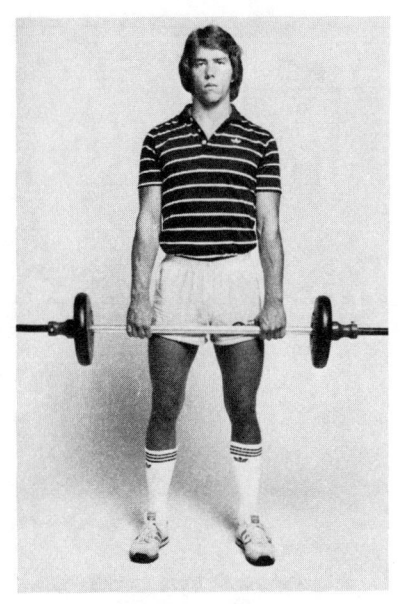

Barbells exercise both arms.

claims as to the effectiveness of their machines — but few of these claims are scientifically substantiated. If you find a machine you enjoy using, stay with it. Whether or not it gives the fastest development it will be effective if you stick with it.

There are several different kinds of machines. The most common device is an isotonic machine using pulleys or levers. The largest manufacturer of these is Universal. Fast growing in popularity are the cam machines produced by Nautilus and Dyna Cam. These are variable-resistance isotonic machines. They use an unsymmetrical cam that varies the load throughout the exercise motion. Another kind is isokinetic machines. They have the smallest share of the market, but seem to be gaining in popularity. Isokinetic equipment uses hydraulic systems, or governors, to control the speed of movement.

If you are unfamiliar with a piece of weight equipment, learn how to use it properly. Written instructions are rarely found in a weight room so you will probably have to seek information from someone there who is knowledgeable. This is especially true with the more sophisticated equipment. For example, to use several pieces of Nautilus equipment, you must position the seat so that the axis of rotation of the machine coincides with your axis of

60   STRENGTH EXERCISES

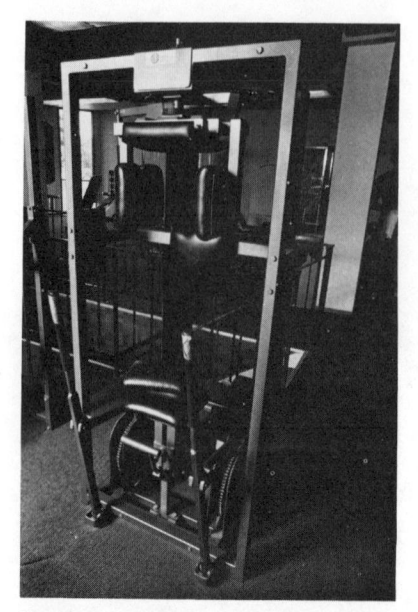

Nautilus equipment is at better gyms.

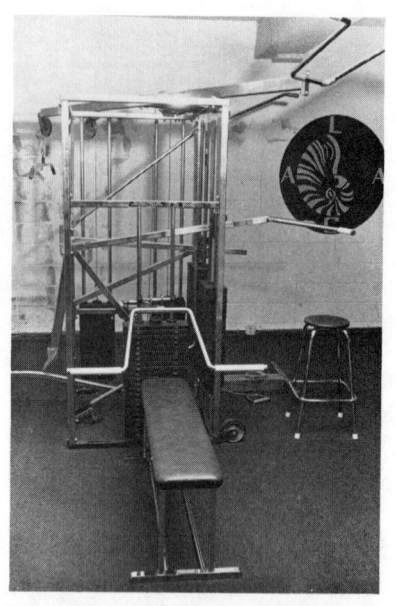

Universal equipment is popular and well-known.

rotation or joint, in the exercise. The only way to find the best seating position is to have someone on the staff assist you.

Because weight machines are expensive, most facilities do not have all the sets of equipment needed to exercise all the body's muscles; therefore, you should augment the machine workout with free weights.

There is no doubt that machines are effective in developing strength; however, there is a continuing debate over how beneficial that strength is for sports or fitness. The attractiveness of using machines is that someone who is not a weightlifter can improve and the possibility of injury is slight.

One piece of weight equipment that is often not found in a weight facility is an iron boot. Iron boots and ankle weights allow you to do a variety of exercises for the ankles and legs that are important to a number of sports. You can easily make a set of ankle weights, or purchase them at a sporting goods store. To make a set, buy 25 pounds of lead shot and then make four bags, out of denim, that will lay across the top of your foot. Divide the shot into 2½, 5, 7½ and 10 pounds and fill the four cloth bags.

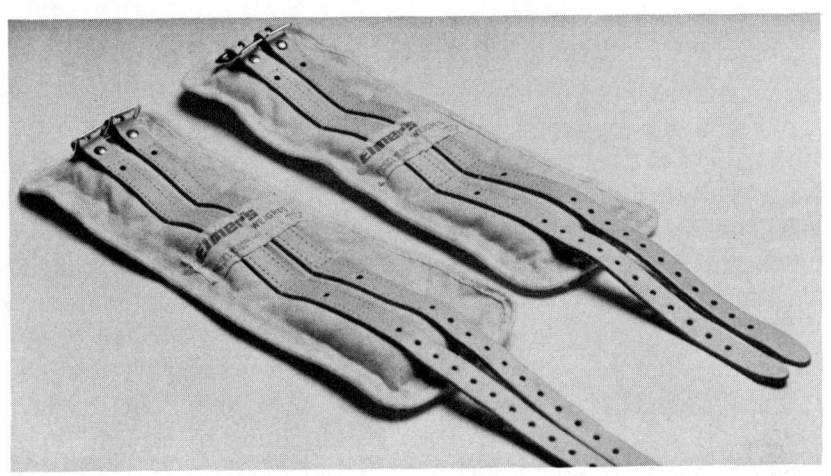

Ankle weights increase resistance.

Add straps — Velcro fasteners are nice — and you have a set of ankle weights.

Whichever equipment you use — or maybe you will not use any — the principle and techniques of strength training still apply.

GROUP 1: MOTIONS OF THE LOWER LEG

Motions of the lower leg are controlled by muscles along the upper leg: the quadriceps and hamstring groups. These groups, each composed of several muscles, extend (quadriceps) and flex (hamstrings) the lower leg through the largest joint in the body, the knee.

Muscle strength in the quadriceps and hamstrings is essential to provide stability for the knee and to prevent injuries to that joint. Performance in most sports, whether endurance or power sports, requires muscle strength in this pair.

Because of the very large size of these muscles, it is a good practice to start a workout with exercises for them. The quadriceps are the stronger of the two muscles and the ones emphasized in most sports; nonetheless, the hamstring should generally be about 60 percent as strong as the quadriceps.

1a Leg Extension

Leg extensor muscles are located along the front of the thigh. There are two types of exercises to strengthen these muscles. In the first, resistance is applied to the front of the lower leg at the ankle and the leg is extended to a straight-leg position. This exercise is most often done on a leg extension/flexion machine, either of an isotonic or isokinetic type. It is one of the best exercises for any sport that requires running or leg strength and is prescribed for rehabilitation of many knee injuries.

When doing leg extensions isotonically, move at a steady pace throughout the exercise. It is common to see people jerk the weights during the initial motion of the exercise — the weights continue upward with little added effort at the other angles of extension. Thus, the only strength gained is at the initial angle. To counteract this tendency, pause at the maximum extension for a full second before lowering the weights. Resist the fall of the weights so that you will work on both extension and contraction. If the weight equipment does not have restraining belts to help isolate the motion, hold onto the bench you're sitting on by extending your arms behind you for a brace.

The same exercise can be done without a machine by using either an iron boot or ankle weights. Iron boots are available at some facilities. At home you can use a large boot to which you tie weights, bricks for example. An easier method, though, is to use ankle weights.

The second type of leg-extension exercise is known as the squat and variations of the squat. To do squats with barbells, keep your head up, back arched and your feet shoulder-width apart. With the bar resting on your shoulders and held in both hands, bend your knees until your thighs are parallel to the floor and hold this position for several seconds. Then drive with your legs to push yourself upward, returning to your starting position.

There are many horror stories of people injuring their knees while doing squats. Undoubtedly some of the stories are true, but almost all of those accidents could have been avoided. Squats are good exercises if done properly. Lower yourself below the point where your thighs are parallel to the floor and you jeopardize your knees. To prevent this, place a chair behind you; it will stop you from going too low. To give you better stability, stand with your heels on a 2-by-4 and your toes on the floor.

If you want to do deeper, full squats, first ensure that your knees are flexible throughout the full range of motion. Do the exercise with only a bar across your shoulders. Over a several-week period slowly add weight. Always make sure that you squat slowly, in control.

Leg-press machines work nearly the same muscles as do squats. Of course, they remove the requirement for balance and do not

Strength Exercises 63

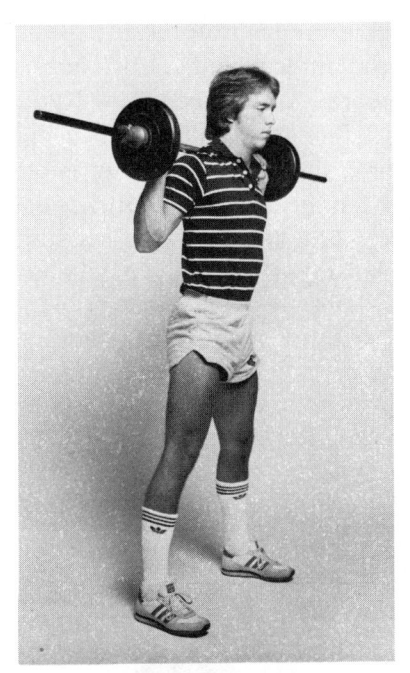

Begin the squat standing.

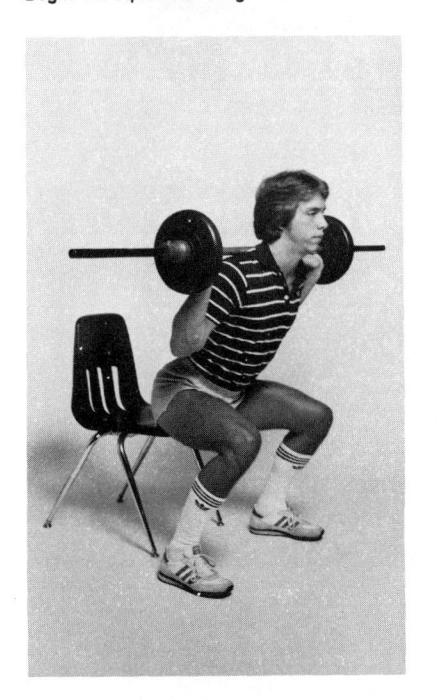

Now bend at the knees.

Use a chair for safety.

force both legs to contribute equally. At an isotonic leg press, position the seat so that you start with your legs bent at a 90° angle. The balls of your feet should be squarely on the pedals and you should be seated with your back flat in the chair. When using heavy weights, anything approaching or exceeding your body weight, you will need to hold yourself in the chair with both hands.

Another variation of this exercise is the stepup. Choose a step height so that when the foot is on the step, the thigh is parallel to the floor. For people taller than five feet, a 12-inch step is adequate. An 18- or 20-inch step can be used for people taller than six

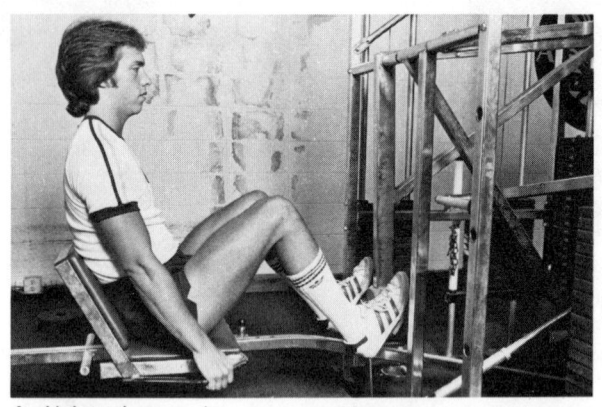

A Universal gym leg press machine.

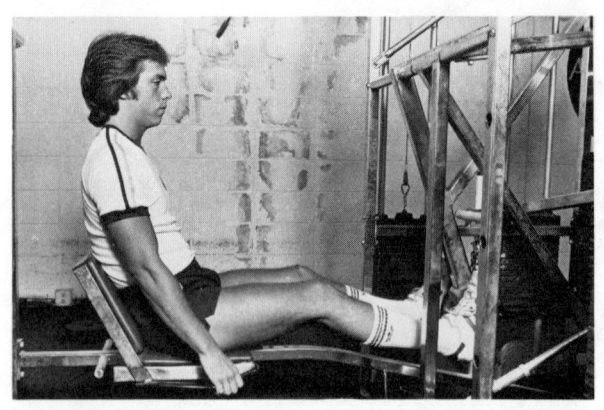

Extend the legs in one motion.

feet. When you step up, place your other foot on the step, too. Use one leg to lead for the full count of repetitions before switching legs.

To stretch the leg extensors, stand, and place one hand on a wall for support. With the other hand, grasp the toes of the foot on the same side and gently pull the toes upward toward your buttocks. Hold a comfortable position for 20 seconds and then switch sides.

1b Leg Flexion

Flexion of the lower leg is done almost entirely by muscles in the hamstring group. These muscles are along the back of the upper leg. Without weights it is difficult to exercise this muscle. The isotonic leg machine, used for leg extensions, also can be used for hamstring curls. Remember to pull smoothly and strive for full contraction. Your foot should touch or almost touch your buttocks when your leg is at maximum contraction. Rest your chin, not your cheek, on the bench to ensure that you get a balanced workout.

You can use ankle weights to do hamstring curls. Attach the weight to your foot and flex your leg. This can be done while either standing or lying on your stomach. If done while standing, the maximum effort will be required when the leg is bent at a $90°$ angle. While lying down, the maximum effort will be exerted at the smallest angles of contraction, when the leg is nearly flat on the floor; no effort will be exerted when the leg is beyond a $90°$ bend. If you are going to use ankle weights for the exercise, you should vary your position in order to work the hamstrings at all angles.

There is one way to strengthen the hamstrings without weights. Lie on your back and bend your knees. Draw your feet, along the ground, toward your buttocks. You can apply more resistance by putting weight on your legs and raising your buttocks off the ground. You can ruin a carpet doing this, so practice it on the beach or on a hard floor.

The hamstring muscles should be about 60 percent as strong as the leg extensors. If they are much weaker than this, they could be injured while running.

66 STRENGTH EXERCISES

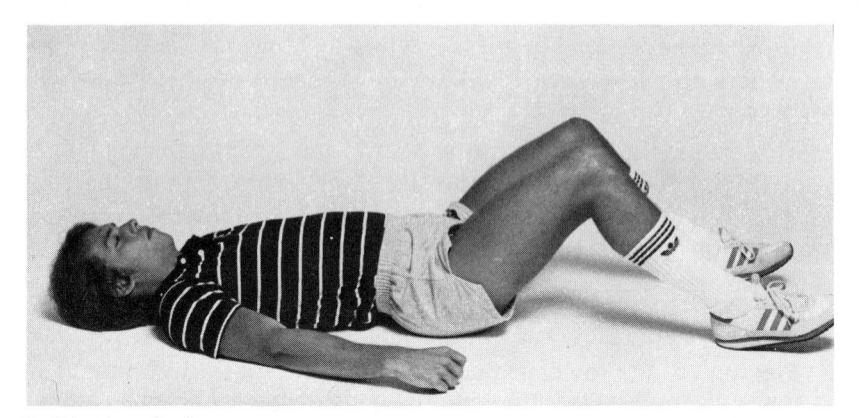

Push hard on the floor.

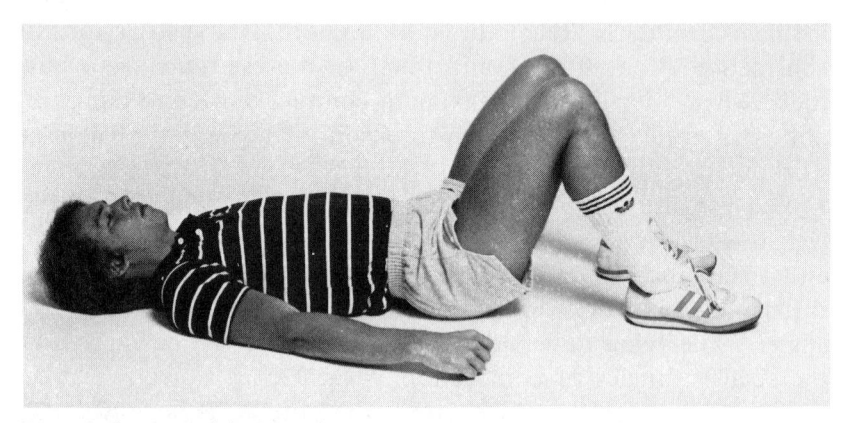

Draw the feet toward the buttocks.

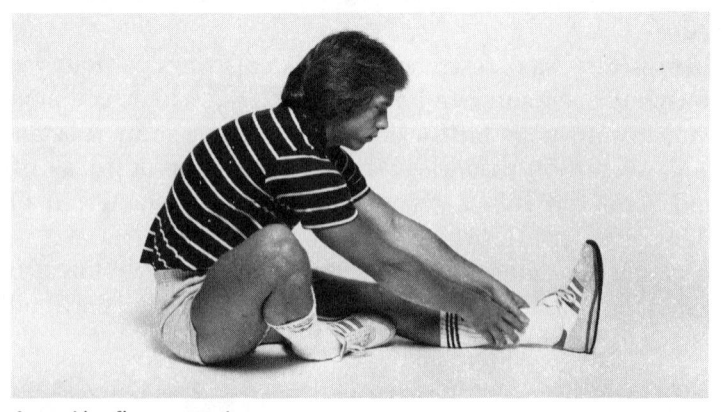

A good leg flexor stretch.

There are many ways to stretch the leg flexors. One of the best is to sit on the floor on your back with your legs straight at the knee. Spread your legs so they are at right angles (90°) to each other. Bend the right leg at the knee and place the sole of the right foot alongside the left knee. Bend at the waist and with both hands reach toward your left foot. Make sure the toes of the foot are pointing upward and not out to the side. When you find a comfortable position, hold it for 20 seconds. Repeat the stretch for the right leg.

MOTIONS OF THE UPPER LEG

Motions of the upper leg are driven by the 22 muscles of the hip. This grouping of muscles is the largest mass of muscles in the body. There are four principal motions: 1) Extension − pulling the legs to the rear, bringing them toward the plane of the trunk. Hyperextension occurs when they are pulled back, beyond the plane of the trunk. 2) Flexion − pulling the legs forward, away from the body plane, as in kicking a ball. 3) Abduction − pulling a leg outward, away from the centerline of the body. 4) Adduction − pulling the leg toward the centerline. Two additional motions are inward and outward rotation of the leg; however, the abductor and adductor muscles are responsible for rotation and so separate rotator exercises are not given. Extension and flexion exercises are included in Group 2 and abduction and adduction exercises are in Group 3.

GROUP 2: EXTENSION AND FLEXION OF THE UPPER LEG

2a Extension

Extension of the hip is accomplished principally by the large muscles in the buttocks (gluteus maximus) and secondarily by the hamstrings along the back of the upper leg. Hip extensors, especially the gluteus maximus, get little exercise, except in a workout. For that reason the muscle loses tone and can be the preferential place for storage of body fat. Gaining muscle strength can improve appearance as well as balance the strong hip flexor muscles.

Hip-extension exercises require the use of a table or weight-room equipment. Rest your chest on the table and grasp the sides of the table or the foot braces on the back extension station. Raise both legs together, and hold them as straight and as high as you can. Then lower them slowly until the toes touch the floor. Do not do the exercise so quickly that the legs are accelerated in the

68 STRENGTH EXERCISES

first few degrees of movement, which results in no effort being expended beyond that point.

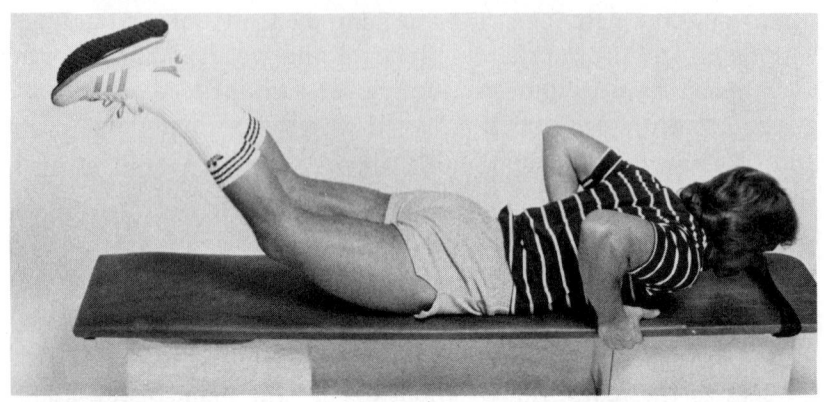

Lower the legs slowly.

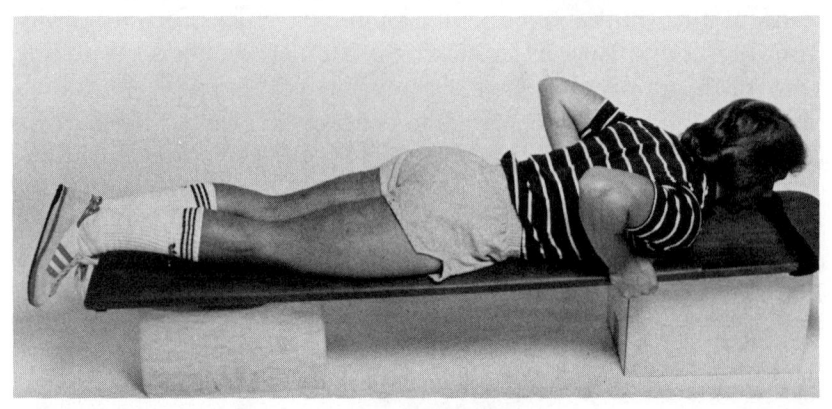

This works the hip extensors.

An alternative exercise, which I call the swimmer's kick, is to pull one leg up and let the other down, instead of both legs going in the same direction.

Nautilus has an excellent machine, the hip and back machine, to work the hip extensor. When using this equipment, brace yourself in position by holding the handles and keeping your arms locked at the elbows. Do the exercise slowly but without rest between repetitions.

If you do not have a table, you can do two other exercises. Hold onto a railing or a doorknob that is waist-high. Bend at the waist so that your back is horizontal and then steady yourself by

Strength Exercises 69

holding onto the railing. Raise one leg behind you as high as possible, keeping it straight. Complete the desired repetitions with one leg before starting on the other.

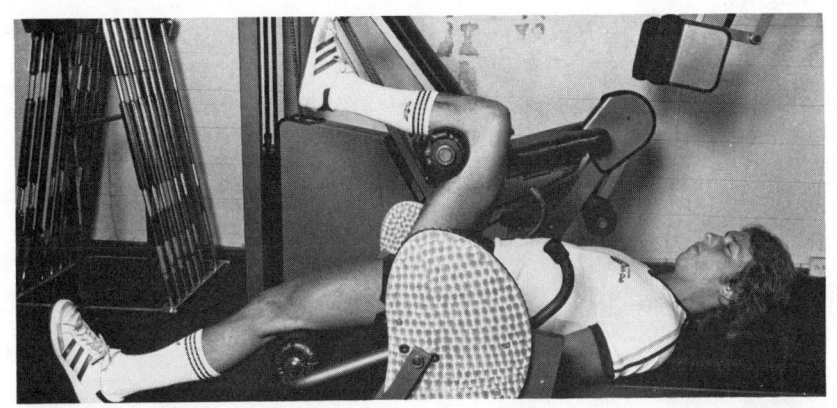

Nautilus hip and back machine.

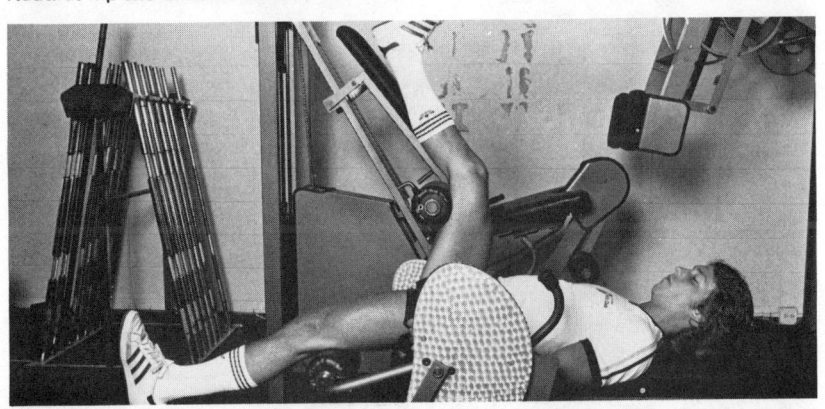

Start with bent knee.

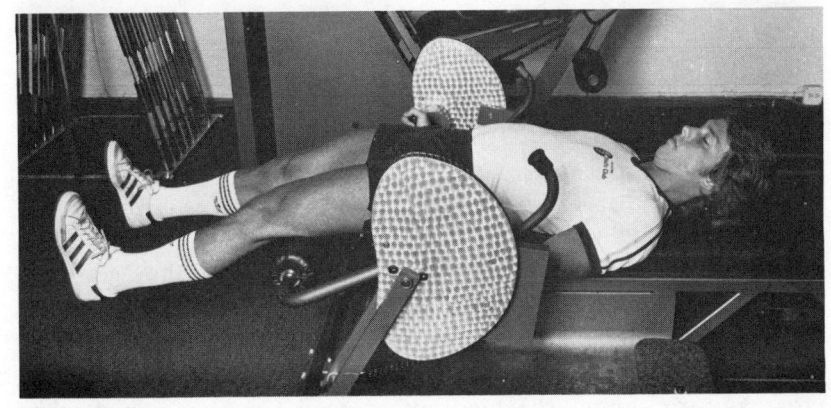

Push leg forward.

A variation of this is to stand erect while facing a wall and then to raise one leg behind you. Again, keep the leg straight at the knee. To increase resistance in any of these exercises, use ankle weights.

To stretch the hip extensors you'll need to lie on your back. Now bend one leg and grasp it with both hands just below the knee. Pull the leg up to your chest until you feel a stretching sensation in your buttocks and lower back.

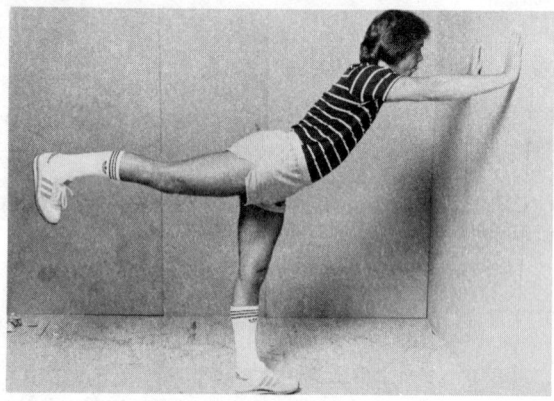

Lean on the wall and raise the leg.

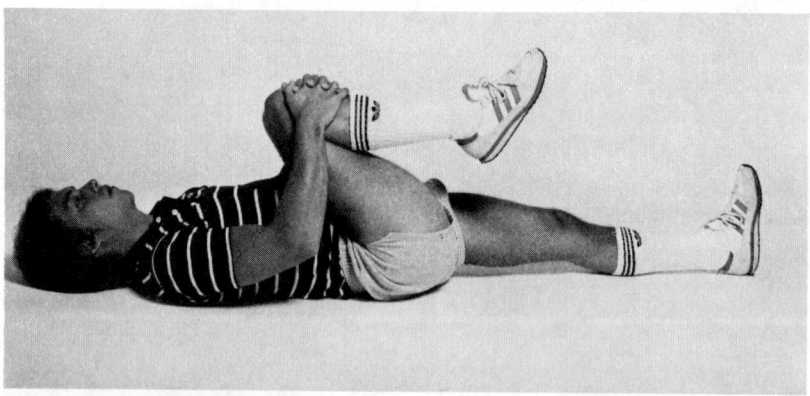

Pull with both hands on the knee.

2b Flexion of the Hip

Hip flexors are usually strong muscles, because they get exercise in many types of workouts. For instance, when most people do situps they are exercising the hip flexors more than the abdominal muscles. Except for application to specific sports (for example, cross-country skiing) the hip flexors need less attention than do

Strength Exercises 71

most other muscle groups. In fact, I do not recommend you doing these exercises except for a few sports. An unbalanced development of the hip flexor muscles can lead to back pain.

Exercises of the hip flexors are straight-leg raises of one type or another and full situps. The most common exercise is the double leg raise while lying with your back on the floor. Raise both legs, keeping the knees straight, until the hips rise off the floor, then lower them slowly.

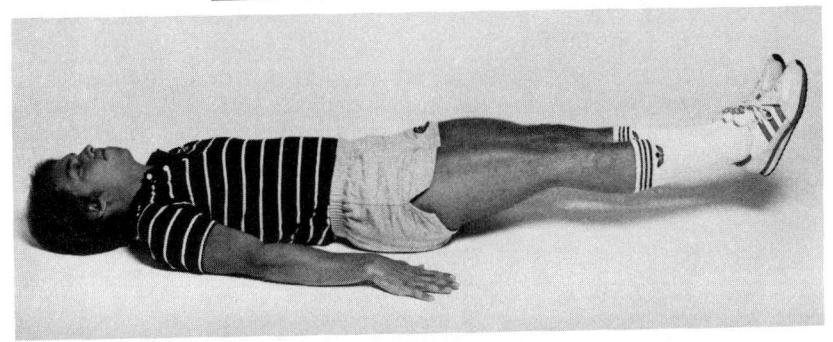

Leg raises work the hip flexors.

Leg raises can also be done while holding onto or hanging from a chinup bar. In the former, raise one thigh as high as possible while standing on the other leg. Add ankle weights to increase the resistance.

While hanging from a bar raise both legs, with straight knees, as high as possible. It is helpful to have a partner steady you during these exercises. Leg raise exercises can strain the muscles in the lower back. If you choose to do these, be careful and stop if you develop back pain.

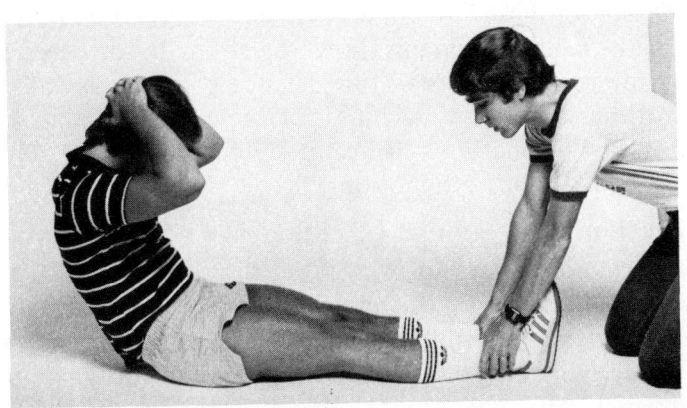

Straight leg situps work the hip flexors.

Straight leg situps, or situps with the feet held down, work the hip flexors more than the abdominal muscles. Also, straight leg situps place a large stress on the back. To do situps for hip flexor development, bend the knees slightly and anchor the feet so they cannot rise or move. Hold your hands behind your head and then sit up, touching the elbow of one arm to the opposing knee. Repeat the situp, this time touching the opposite elbow and knee.

Start from a kneeling position to stretch the hip flexors in this exercise. Place your right foot on the floor in front of you and your left knee on the floor as far back as is comfortable. Then lean forward without moving either the right foot or left knee. Place your hands on the floor to brace yourself.

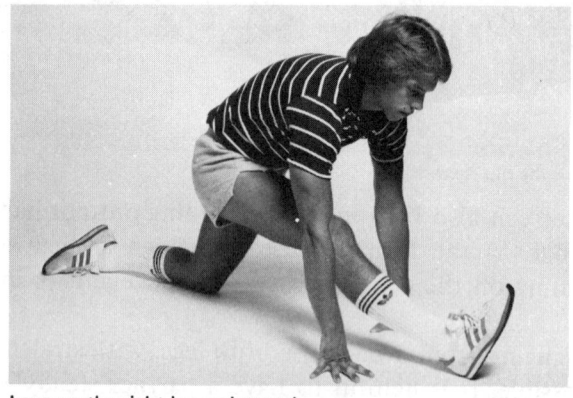

Lean on the right leg and stretch.

GROUP 3: INWARD AND OUTWARD MOVEMENT OF THE LEG

Exercises for these two opposing muscle groups are rarely found in strength-training programs; however, strength is needed in these groups for certain sports — for instance skiing — as well as for general fitness. Exercise machines for these motions exist but are found in few gymnasiums or health clubs. Nautilus has a machine that can be used for both motions.

3a Abduction

Abduction is movement away from the centerline of the body. To exercise muscles in this group, raise one leg directly to the outside as high as possible, keeping the knee straight. This can be done while lying on your side or while standing or lying on an inclined bench. The angle of maximum resistance will be different in each of these positions. Use ankle weights to increase the resistance.

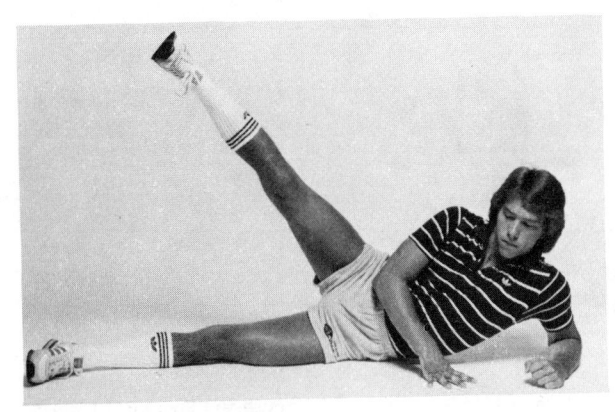

Lift the leg as high as you can.

A variation of this exercise requires a partner. Lie on your back with your legs straight and together. Push your feet away from each other while your partner opposes this motion with his hands. The partner should exert enough pressure so that you slowly overcome his resistance.

To stretch the hip abductors lie on your back with your knees bent and with your hands behind your head. Cross one leg over the knee of the other and use it to pull the second leg down toward the floor. Keep your shoulders flat on the floor.

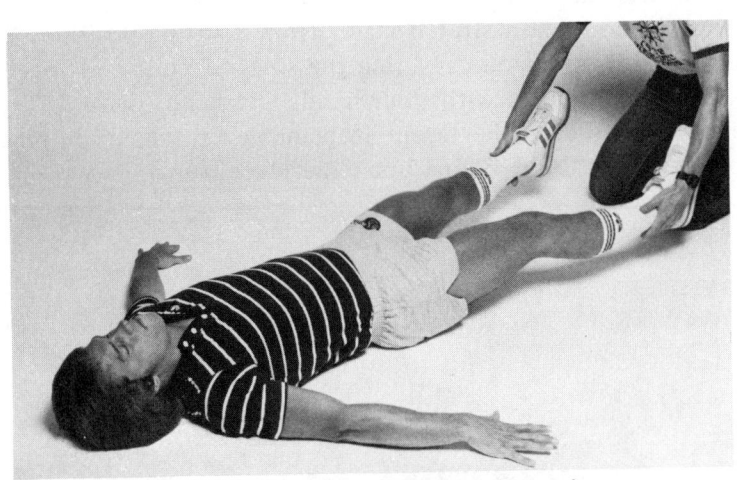

Have your partner push your heels together against resistance.

3b Adduction

Strengthening the muscles that bring your legs in toward the centerline is more difficult. Either you or your partner must supply the resistance. If you are without a partner, sit on the floor

74 STRENGTH EXERCISES

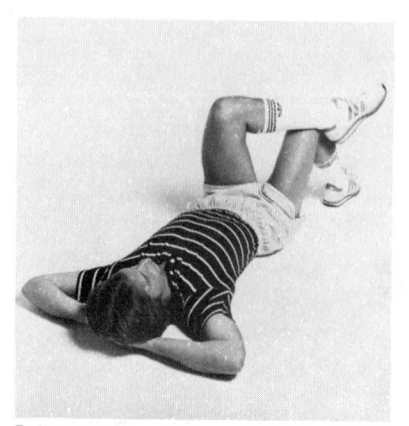

Pull with crossed leg.

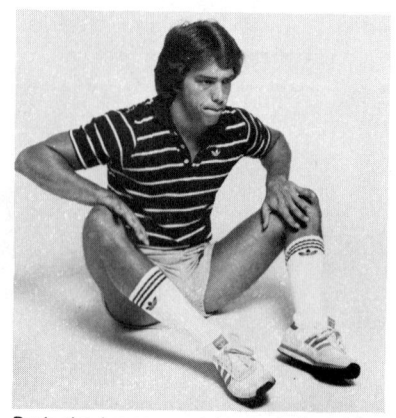

Push the knees apart to work the adduction muscles.

with your legs bent at the knee and your feet flat on the floor. Grasp each knee with your hands. Force your knees apart with your hands while resisting with your adductors; then ease the force applied by your hands so that you can pull your knees together again. This is a very tiring exercise because you are working hard with both arms and legs.

The second adduction exercise is similar to the second abduction exercise. Lie on your back with your legs straight and flat on the floor. Bring your heels together against resistance supplied by your partner who is holding you at your ankles.

The hip adduction stretch starts from a sitting position. Bend your knees so that you can bring the soles of your feet together. Hold onto your toes with your hands and bend forward. Try to touch your nose to the floor. Stop, however, when you reach a good stretch position, before you experience pain.

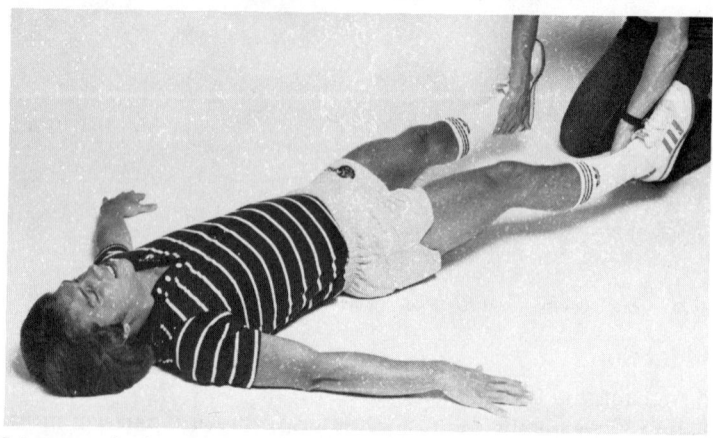

Bring your heels together against resistance.

GROUP 4: MOTIONS OF THE TRUNK

There are three motions of the trunk: flexion, extension, and lateral flexion. A fourth motion, rotation of the trunk relative to the hips, is not included here because the muscles that produce rotation also are used in flexion and lateral flexion.

Aches and pains in the lower back can be avoided by strengthening trunk muscles. Lower-back aches arise from muscle fatigue. The muscles get little exercising day to day, but on occasional weekends they are expected to perform herculean tasks. Weak abdominal muscles contribute to the problem. As a stomach bulge degenerates into a paunch, the back muscles must constantly work to hold the spine erect. To avoid backaches, exercise both the abdominal and back muscles.

4a Trunk extension

Extensors of the trunk lie along the back and pull against the hips to straighten the back. They can pull the back beyond a straight line, arching the back, which is called back hyperextension.

The simplest exercise for the muscles of the lower back is toe touches. With feet close together and knees straight, bend over at the waist as far as you can and then raise your back. Besides strengthening back muscles, this exercise stretches the hamstrings.

To increase resistance, use a barbell. This exercise is called the **straight leg dead lift**. Start with just the bar itself and increase

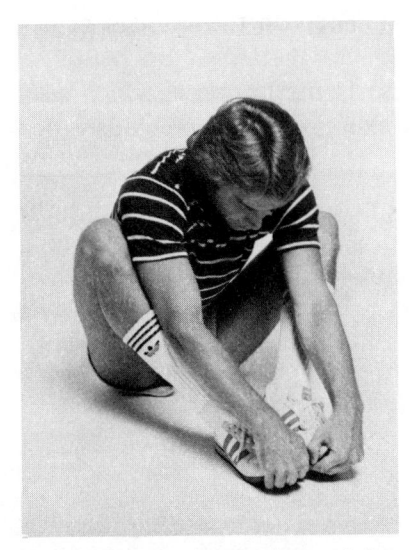

Hip adduction stretch from sitting position.

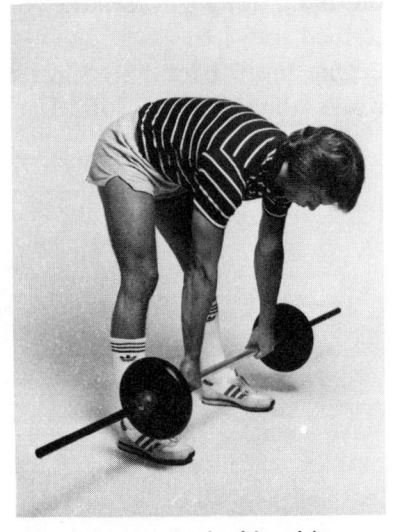

Deadlift is a toe-touch with weight.

resistance very slowly. Because it is easy to exceed the limits of your back muscles, I do not generally recommend this exercise for strength training.

I prefer back extensions. Unfortunately, to do these requires some equipment that is rarely found outside a weight room. Rest your lower stomach on the pad and hold yourself in position by pressing one foot on the pedal and hooking the heel of the other foot under the padded block. With hands behind your head, lower your trunk as far as possible. Raise it up slowly as far as possible and hold the position of maximum extension for a full second. Oppose the force of gravity on both upward and downward motions. Do not accelerate during the early stages of extension so that you fly upward into a hyperextension position. You can easily overstretch your back, but by going slowly you cannot injure your back.

To increase resistance, hold a barbell weight against the back of your neck. Hold it tightly so that it does not bang your head.

If this exercise equipment is not available, there are two other methods that will allow you to do back extensions. The first is to lie stomach down on a sturdy table. Extend your upper body beyond the edge of the table and have a partner hold your legs down. Then do the exercise as described above. The second alternative is to construct a back extension station. Some parcourses have such stations. Construct a narrow table to rest your stomach on and a railing to secure your feet. Then do the exercise as described above.

One more back extension exercise is the hip raise, which also works the hip extensors. Use this exercise if the previously de-

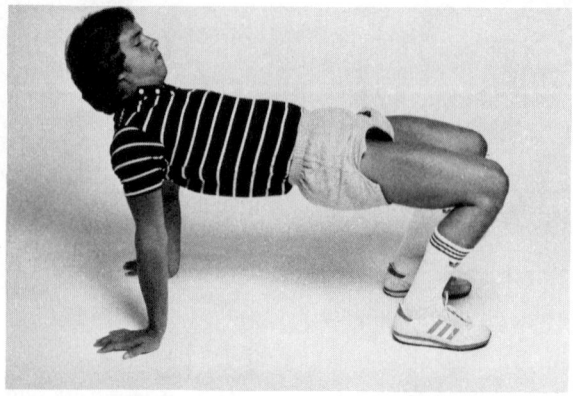

You might call this the crab crawl.

scribed exercises are too difficult. From a sitting position, support your weight on your feet and hands, keeping your knees tightly bent. Then raise your hips so that your thighs and back are in a straight line.

I recommend two stretches for the extensor muscles of the lower back. The first is the old standard—toe touches. Spread your feet shoulder-width apart. Bend at the waist and reach for

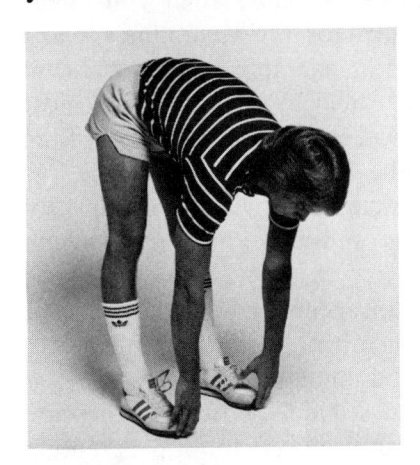

Toe touches are good for the back.

your toes. Of course, it does not matter if you reach them or not, just get a good stretch. As you recover to the upright standing position, bend your knees slightly and this will reduce the stress on your lower back.

The second stretch starts from a cross-legged, sitting position.

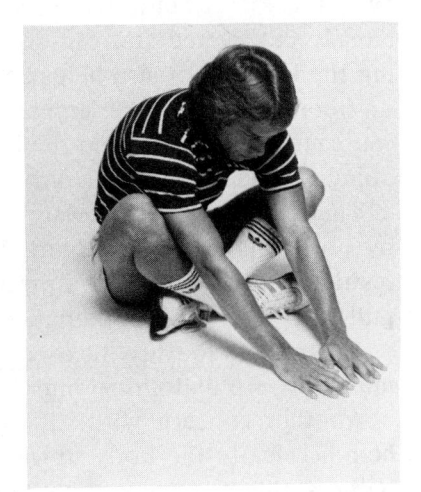

Try to touch your head to the floor.

Bend forward and try to touch your head to the floor in front of you.

If you have a history of back problems, check with a physician before doing any of these exercises.

4b Trunk flexion

Trunk flexion is accomplished largely by the abdominal muscles. To adequately exercise these muscles is harder than you might imagine. In many exercises prescribed for the abdominals, other muscles do much of the exercise. For example, when situps are done with straight legs and with feet held by a strap or bar, most of the work is performed by the hip-flexor muscles instead of the abdominals. The hip flexors pull the hips up relative to the legs while the abdominals pull the trunk up relative to the hips. By watching the motions of trunk, hips and legs, you can see which muscles are doing the most work.

As an experiment, do a set of situps, keeping your knees locked and feet held down by a partner or under a piece of furniture. Feel which muscles, hip flexors or abdominals, tire first.

Granted, hip flexor muscles need strength, but often they are already much stronger than their antagonists, the hip extensors in the buttocks. A large imbalance between this pair of muscle groups can lead to lower-back pain. Also, by allowing the hip flexors to do much of the work in a situp, the abdominals are not getting the workout they need.

One way to help isolate situps to the abdominal muscles is to keep the knees bent. With bent knees the hip flexor muscles are already contracted and can do less to assist the abdominals. Keeping the knees bent also helps keep the back flat on the situp board or floor while you are supine. Otherwise the back arches, which can cause muscle strain in the back while doing situps. Thus, when doing situps always keep your knees bent.

The second way to isolate situps to the abdominal muscles is by not using a foot restraint. When you lock your feet under a restraining belt or under a piece of furniture, the hip flexors can pull your hips up by pulling against your legs. Without a restraint on your feet, the hip flexors cannot be effective—to sit up you must use your abdominal muscles.

Another concern with situps is the use of the head or arms to help accelerate the body upward. Clasping hands behind the head reduces this tendency; however, people will swing their elbows forward to help with the takeoff. This action becomes more prominent as the abdominal muscles tire after a few repetitions. Since the abdominal muscles are most effective at the smallest angles of the exercise, throwing the arms or head forward at the start of the exercise can rob the abdominals of any work. If you tend to do this, try sitbacks instead of situps. From a sitting position with

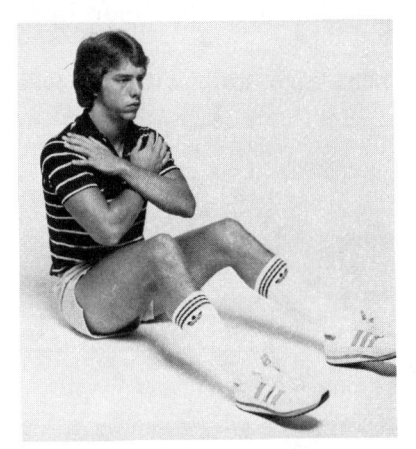

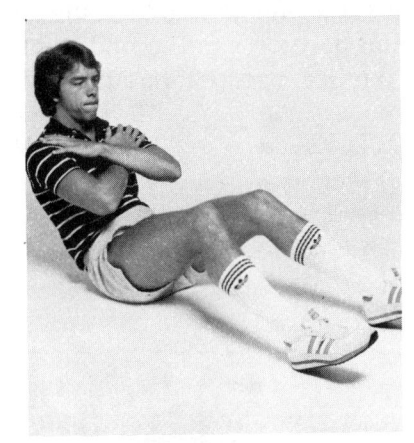

The sitback is opposite of a situp.

Let yourself down slowly.

your hands either behind your head or across your chest, sit back to a supine position while counting slowly to 10. Sit up quickly and repeat.

To increase the exercise resistance, hold a barbell weight behind your head. Or you can increase resistance by doing situps on an inclined board. Start at the bottom position and as your stomach

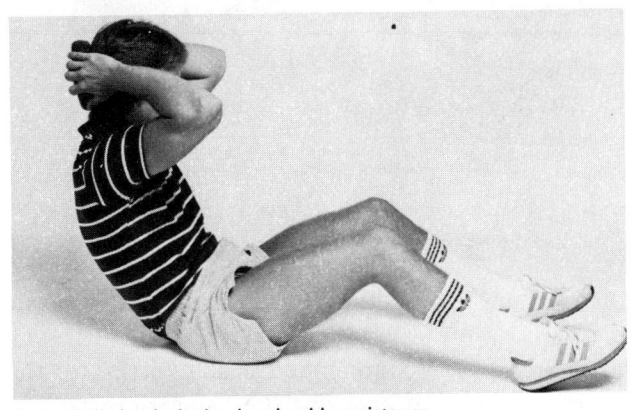

A barbell behind the head adds resistance.

muscles strengthen, increase the angle of the board. Both of these exercises will require that you use a foot restraint.

Full situps are difficult to do with bent knees and with feet flat on the floor without some kind of restraint. An easier exercise from this position is a partial situp or abdominal curl. Clasping your hands behind your head, slowly curl your head and trunk up just far enough so that your shoulder blades are off the floor. Hold this position a full second and slowly uncurl.

I like to do a variation of the bent-knee situp with my feet

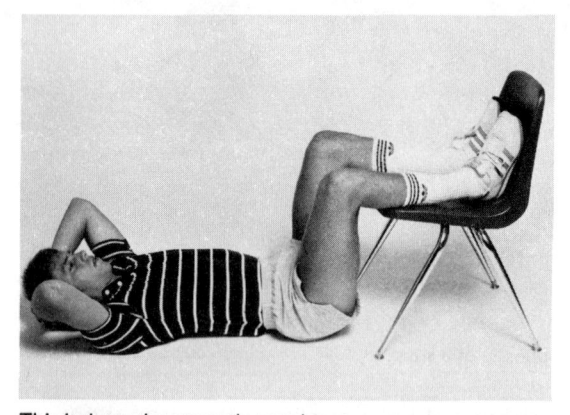

This isolates the stomach muscles.

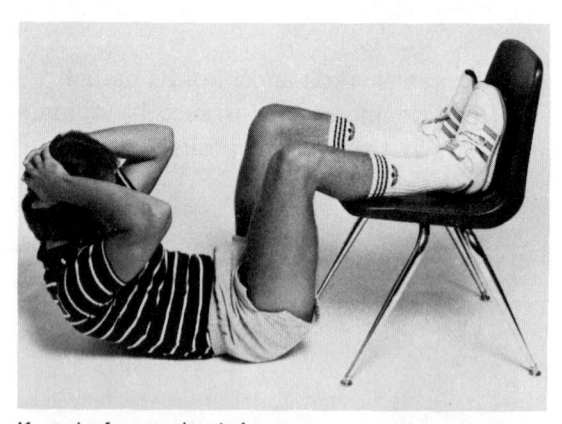

Keep the feet on the chair.

resting on a chair. From this position I do either partial or full situps.

Leg raises are often recommended as an exercise for the abdominals. However, they suffer from the same drawback as regular situps do—they are more exercise for the hip flexors than the

Strength Exercises 81

abdominals. Although the stomach muscles are tense throughout this exercise, they are merely stabilizing the hips. They get isotonic exercise with resistance only when they lift the hips upward and off the floor or situp board. Leg raises should be done through a small arc of motion—from the point where knees meet nose to

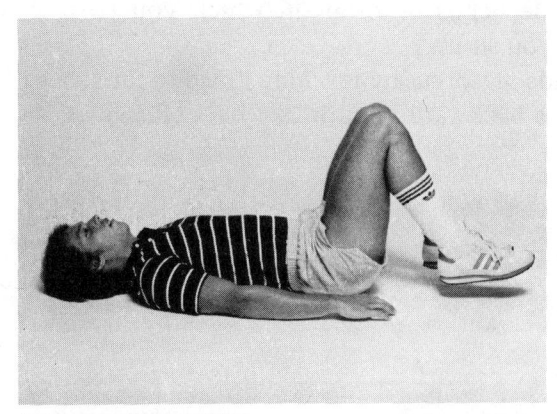

Start at the bent position.

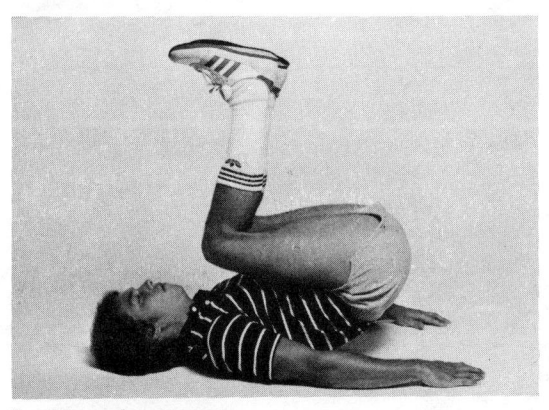

Bend toward your nose.

the point where the hips rest on the floor. An easy way to do this exercise is to keep your knees bent. Your downward motion will stop when your feet hit the floor. To increase the difficulty keep your legs straight at the knees, but stop your downward progress when your hips rest on the floor.

Most of the work done in flexing the trunk or sitting up is done by the abdominals. These muscles can be seen in well-conditioned lean people as the two bands of rippled muscles extending from the ribs to the waistline. However, assistance in trunk flexion is

82 STRENGTH EXERCISES

provided by the oblique abdominal muscles. These muscles connect to the lower four to eight ribs and to the hips. Their oblique position allows them to cause lateral flexion and trunk rotation as well as flexion. The obliques receive some exercise when the abdominals are worked. Additional strengthening can be achieved by doing side bends or situps in which you twist your body to one side as you sit up.

Side bends are done by reaching down to the side without either a forward or backward bend in the back. Reach as low as possible

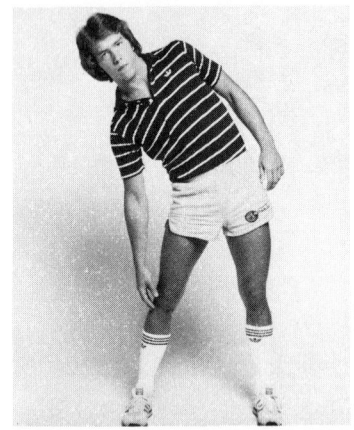

Bend to the right.

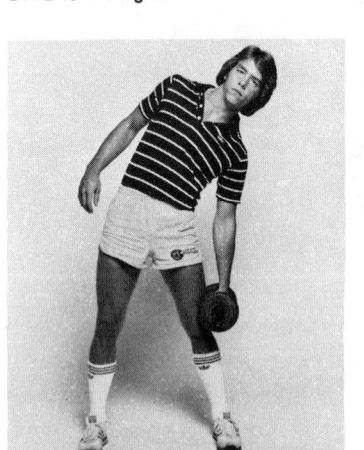

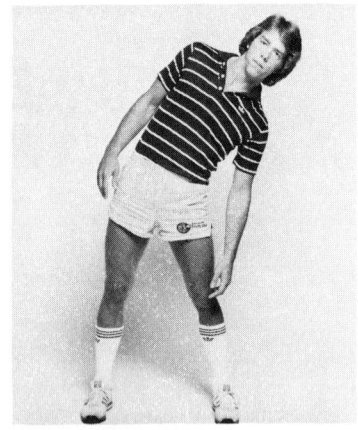

Now bend to the left.

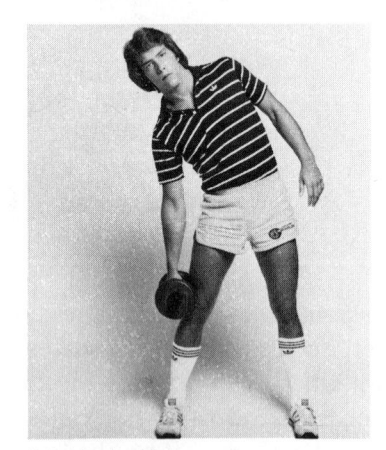

Weights add to the stretch.

Bend both sides.

and then return to a standing position. To maintain your balance, spread your feet a little wider then shoulder-width. Once you have done this exercise a few times, increase the resistance by holding a dumbbell in one hand and bending to the side with the dumbbell. After a set of exercises on one side, switch the dumbbell to the other hand and repeat.

To stretch your trunk flexors, plus several other muscles, lie on the floor on your back. **Stretch your arms out above your head**

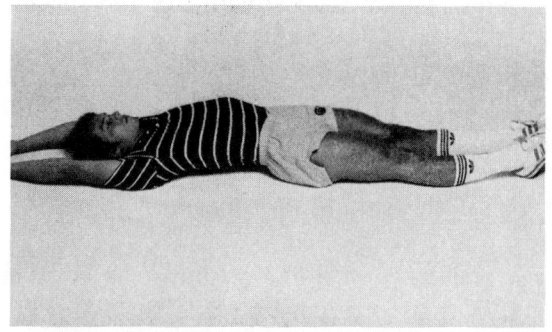

A whole-body stretch for the trunk.

and stretch your toes the opposite direction.

GROUP 5: MOVEMENT OF THE LOWER ARM

Most people associate strength training with exercising the muscles that move the lower arm. The size of a person's biceps and triceps are often taken as a measure of overall strength. For these

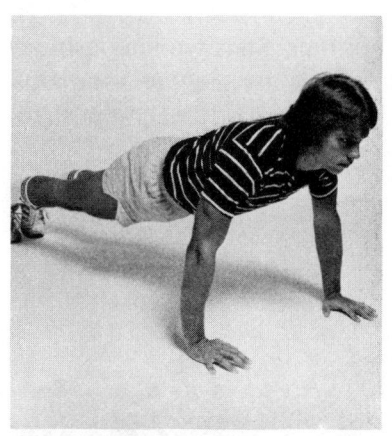

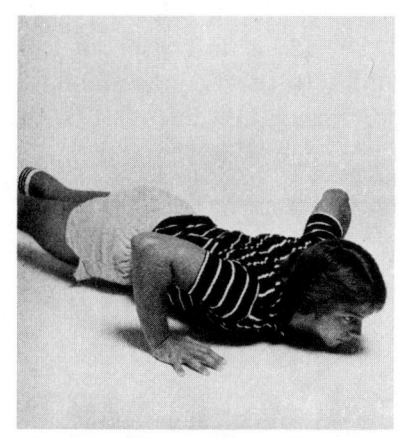

Start the pushup with arms straight.   Lower your chin to the floor.

reasons people who weight train often overindulge themselves in exercising their biceps and triceps, at the expense of other, less glamorous muscles.

The elbow restricts motions of the lower arm. The permitted

motions, extension and flexion, are largely controlled by the triceps and the biceps. The action of these muscles are easy to isolate and there are several exercises for each.

5a Arm extension

The most popular exercise for the lower-arm extension is the pushup. Depending partly on the width of the spacing of hands, pushups strengthen several other muscles. With a wide spacing, the adductors of the upper arm, the pectorals, do much of the work. These muscles, located in the chest, pull the upper arms in toward the centerline of the body. Narrow hand spacing favors strength development in the triceps. Part of the deltoid muscle (which is located on top of the shoulder—upper arm joint) also assists in doing pushups.

The exercise resistance in doing pushups can be changed easily. This is unusual in that for most exercises that do not use weights it is difficult to increase or decrease resistance. The standard pushup starts from a position in which the body is supported on the toes and the palms of the hands. The back is held straight. Feet are together and the hands are shoulder-width apart, and the fingers point ahead of you. The body is lowered by bending the elbows, until the chest touches the floor. Then it is pushed back up. The head should be up, not facing the floor, and the elbows should be kept close to the sides.

To reduce the resistance, do knee pushups. Start from a position similar to that for the standard pushup but use the knees for support instead of the toes. In this position the body weight pushed

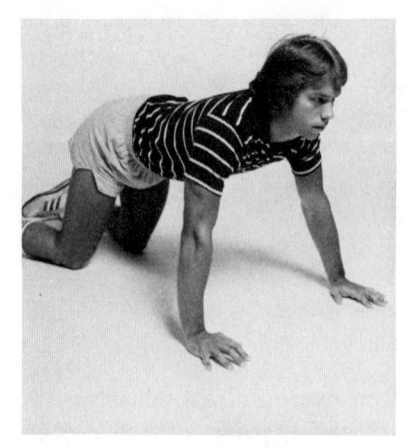

Knee pushups reduce resistance.

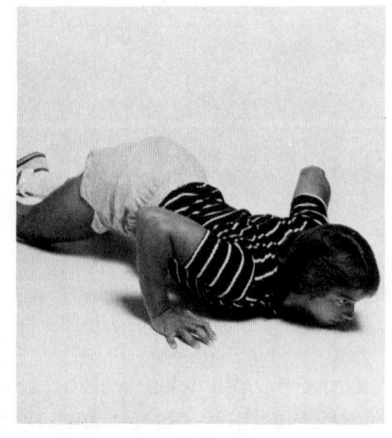

Arm extensors get a break.

by the arm extensors is reduced. Another way to reduce the resistance is to place your hands on an elevated surface, like a sofa or chair. If this is still too difficult, start out by doing pushups while leaning against a wall.

To increase the resistance, do standard pushups with the feet elevated. If you continue to increase the elevation you can do

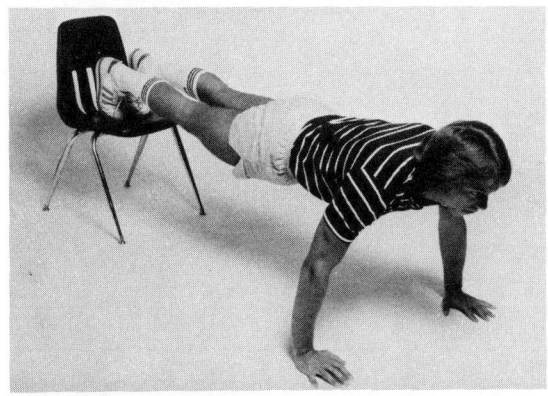

Rest your feet on a chair.

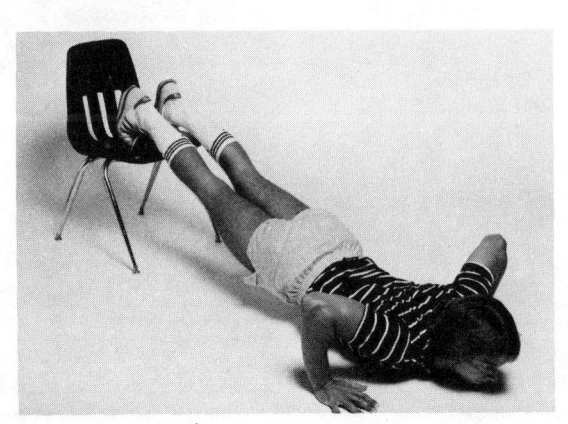

This pushup is tougher.

handstand pushups. This exercise also involves the deltoids, which elevate the upper arm.

If you want to emphasize the muscles in the chest (pectorals) while doing pushups, use a wider hand stance. Also rotate your hands outward.

Another exercise that does not require weights is dips. Dips are done either at a dipping station or on parallel bars. Starting from a position of supporting your weight on straight arms, bend the elbows until the upper arm is horizontal. Then push up to the

86 STRENGTH EXERCISES

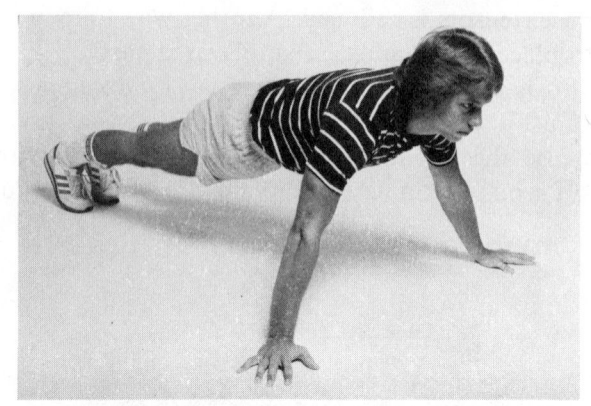

Use a wide stance to work chest muscles.

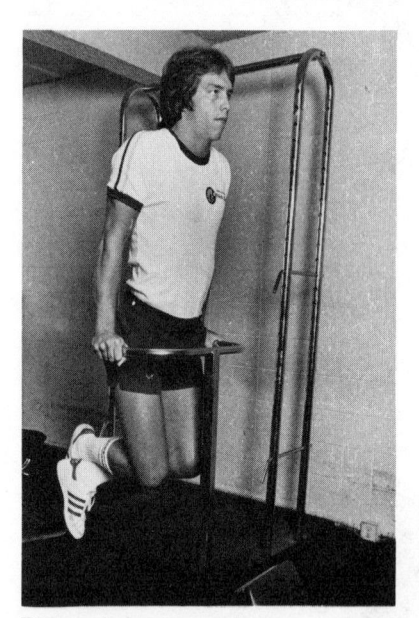

Dips work the arm extensors. Let yourself drop as low as you can.

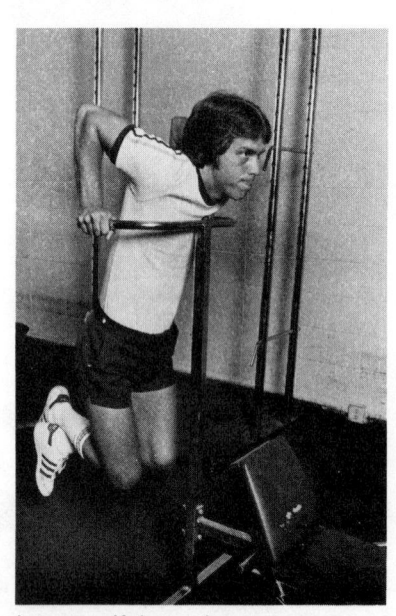

starting position. Work on eliminating any body motion backward or forward.

An easier version can be done using two stable chairs on which you prop your arms. Let your feet rest on the floor or on a third chair in front of you. Lower yourself as far as is comfortable—then push up.

By using weights there are even a greater number of exercises for the arm extensors; the bench press is the most popular. It is similar to pushups except that in doing the bench press you push the resistance away from you, instead of pushing yourself away

Strength Exercises 87

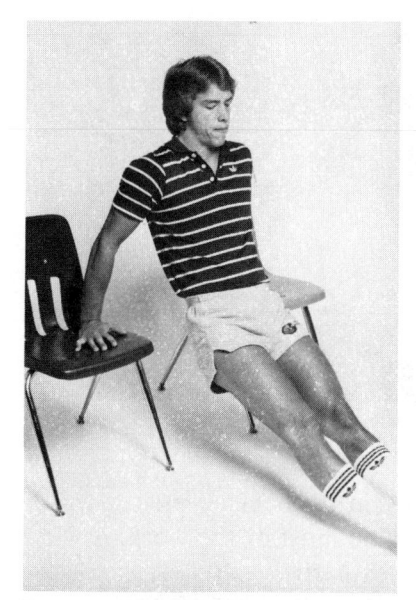

Try dips with two chairs.

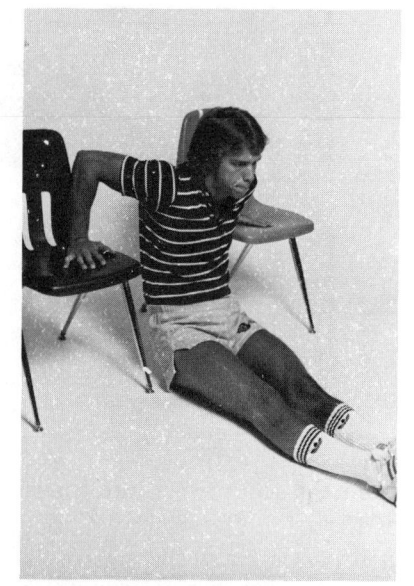

Extend the legs forward.

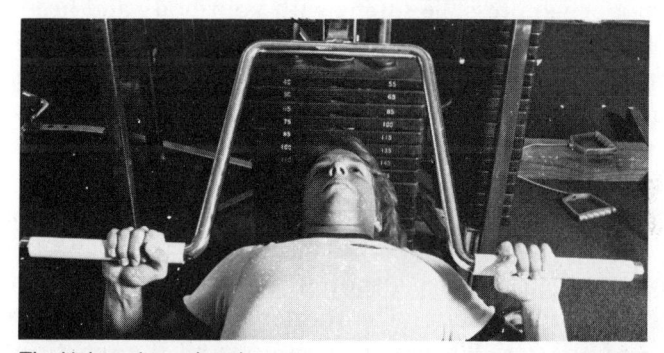

The Universal gym bench press.

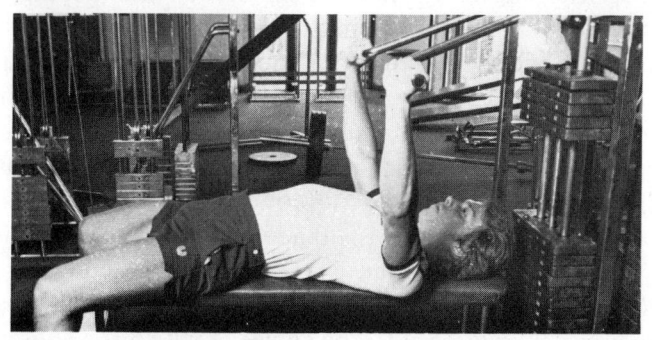

Push the weight away from you.

88 STRENGTH EXERCISES

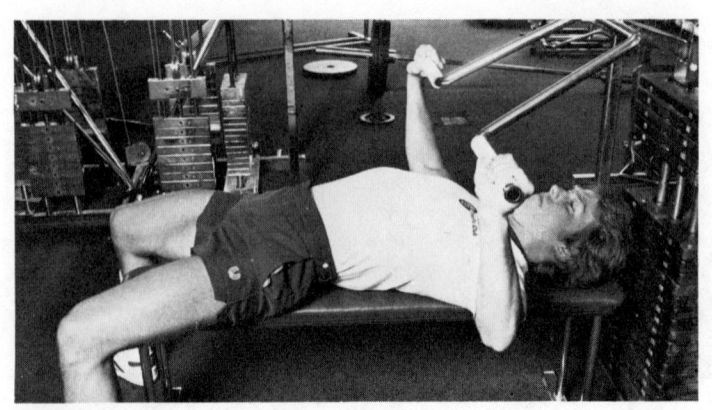

Change your grip to work different muscles.

from the floor. Just like for pushups, in the bench press the width of the grip determines which muscles do most of the work. A wide grip is good for the pectorals while a narrow grip better isolates the arm extensors.

To do a bench press, lie supine with your body and head resting on the bench. If you are shorter than 5 ft. 4 in., you may be more comfortable by putting your feet flat on the bench, knees bent. This position ensures that you do not arch your back. Taller people should put their feet flat on the floor. You should not press down with your feet while doing the exercise. If you are using a weight machine, you will start from a flexed position. Exhale as you push up.

Using a barbell requires a spotter. For very heavy weights two spotters may be necessary. The spotter is used to help at the start and end of the set. When you have done all the repetitions you can, the spotter assists by grabbing the barbell and helping you return it to the rack. If ever left in the embarrassing situation of not being able to move the bar off your chest and not having a spotter, roll the bar to your waist. Sit up and then roll it off your legs, onto the bench.

A common error made in bench pressing is that of not exercising through the full range of motion. In an effort to squeeze out a few extra repetitions, there is a tendency to stop before the position of full contraction is met. The exercise is much easier if you do not lower the weights the entire distance; however, the benefits of the exercise accrue only to the angles at which the exercise was performed. Doing bench presses through half the range of motion is doing half the exercise. The range of motion should be from a position in which elbows are locked to the lowest comfortable position.

The military press is done from a vertical instead of horizontal position. It can be done either standing or sitting. The seated position helps isolate the exercise to arm extensors (triceps) and abductors, or elevators of the upper arm (deltoid muscles). If you do

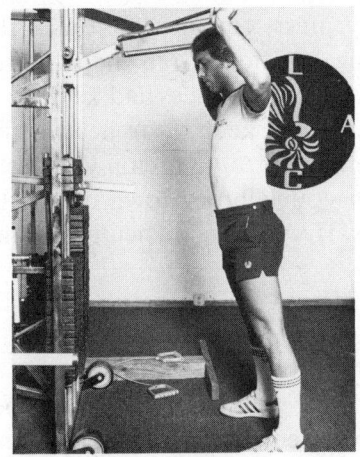

Standing military press.

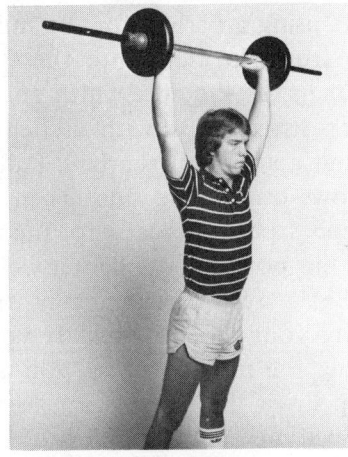

Avoid doing ballistics.

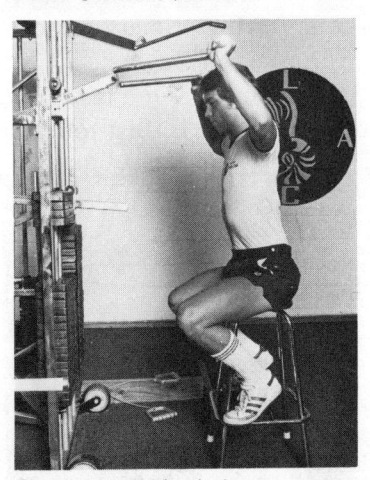

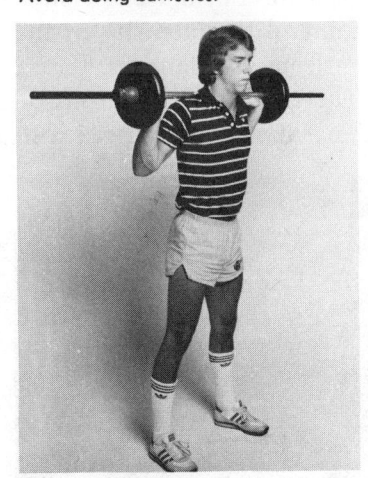

The sitting position isolates arm muscles.

Try varying your grip.

a standing military press, be careful not to bend your back or legs, either of which will help accelerate the weights upward, thus diminishing the isolation. The deltoids are the muscles that elevate the arms from the hanging position at the sides to an overhead position. Basketball players should have well-developed deltoids because they must continually hold their arms up on defense and offense. I recommend this exercise to strengthen both the triceps and deltoids.

To do the military press, grasp the bar with an overhand grip. Press upward as you exhale. Keep your feet shoulder-width apart, your legs straight, and your feet flat on the floor. To do the military press from a seated position you need a sturdy bench that is hip high.

If using a barbell for the military press, you must first raise the bar from the floor into the starting position. Grab the bar with your hands shoulder-width apart. Bend your knees and keep your back straight, or with a slight arch, and keep your head erect. Stand up with the barbell. Pull the bar up to your chin with your elbows out to the side. Then drop your elbows down under the bar in a position ready for the press. If you have difficulty in gaining this position, use lighter weights.

Be aware of the tendency to accelerate the weights upward by using your legs or back. If you bend your back or knees while doing the military press, you are using those extensor muscles to help drive the weights up. Similarly, if you are up on your toes instead of standing flat-footed you are probably bouncing and using your calf muscles. These extraneous motions reduce the isolation and the intensity of the workout for the primary muscles—the triceps and deltoids.

There are two variations of the military press. One is to lower the bar behind your head instead of in front of it. Just touch the

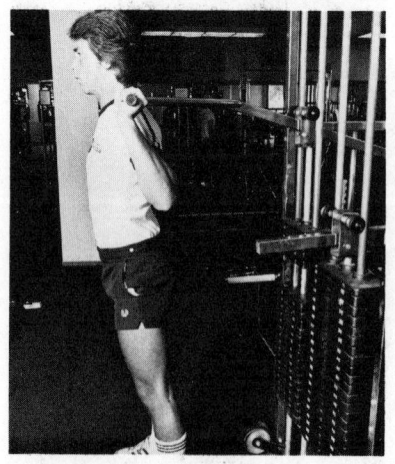

The reverse military press.

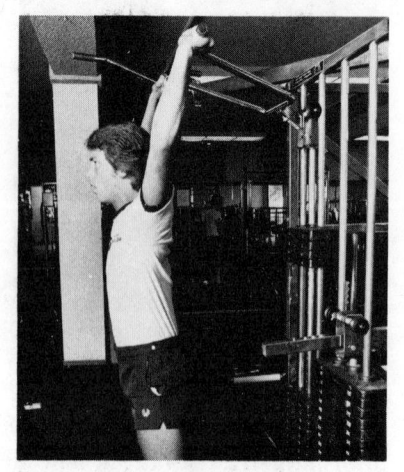

This works the deltoid muscles, posterior side.

bar to the back of your neck and then press upward. If using the military press station on a weight machine, you will have to turn around to face the direction opposite of regular military press. This variation works the posterior part of the deltoid muscle, which is not worked in the other variations.

The second variation is to do a press on an inclined bench. Using a bench makes it more difficult to cheat by using other muscles. This exercise stresses the front part of the deltoids instead of the middle or top part, but otherwise is the same as the military press. Use it for variety in your strength-training program.

All of these press exercises can be done using dumbbells instead of a barbell or a weight machine. Use an overhand grip and alternate pushing one dumbbell while you lower the other.

The differences between using dumbbells, barbells, or a weight machine are small. With a weight machine you can press a heavier

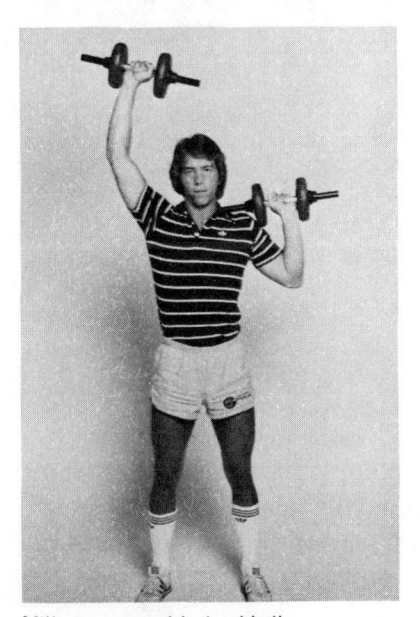

Military press with dumbbells.   Work both arms.

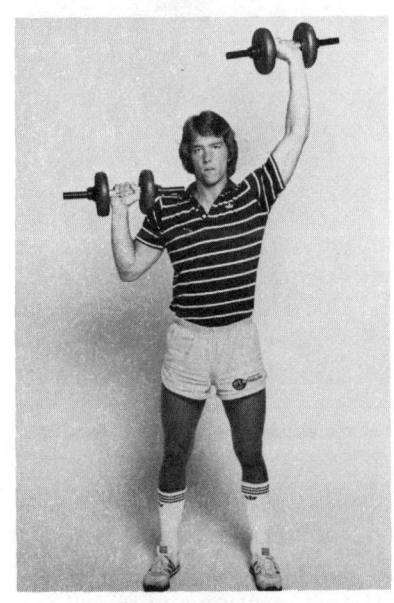

weight because the weights are confined to travel only in one plane of motion. Although you will lift less weight with a barbell, it is a more natural action in that it is unrestricted. If one arm pushes harder than the other, the bar will tilt and you will have to bring it back to the horizontal. One arm can push harder on a weight machine without you knowing it. To overcome this problem, some newer weight machines have been built with split bars so that each arm lifts independently of the other.

Another exercise for the arm extensors is the triceps press. This is done at the lat machine. Grasp the bar with your hands close together in an overhand grip. Keep your elbows tucked in at your sides and without moving your upper arm, press the bar down until your arms are extended.

A similar exercise is the triceps press using a barbell. Rest the bar on your shoulders. Use an overhand grip with your hands closer

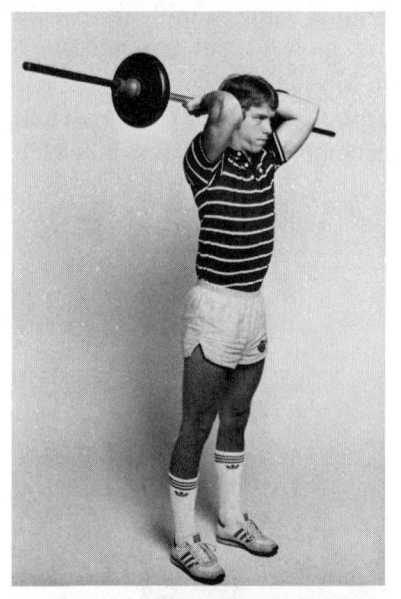

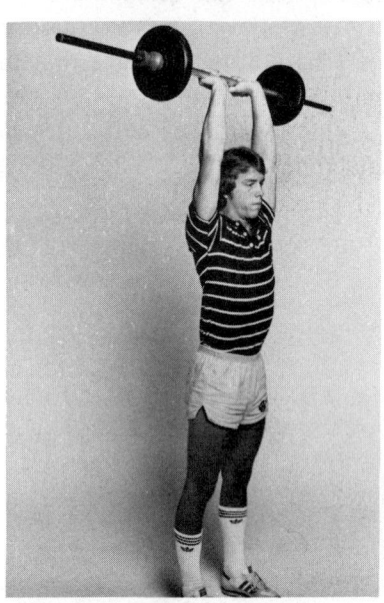

Let the weight down on your shoulders.   Extend the arms, elbows straight.

together than shoulder-width. Keep your elbows close together and pointing forward. Now press the bar upward, over your head with minimum movement of the upper arm. Then return to the starting position and repeat.

On cam-type, variable isotonic machines, the triceps exercise is isolated very well. You position your elbows on a padded block and extend your arms without any other body motion.

To stretch the arm extensors, place the palm of one hand flat on the opposite shoulder blade. The bent arm should pass behind your head. With your free hand pull the elbow downward.

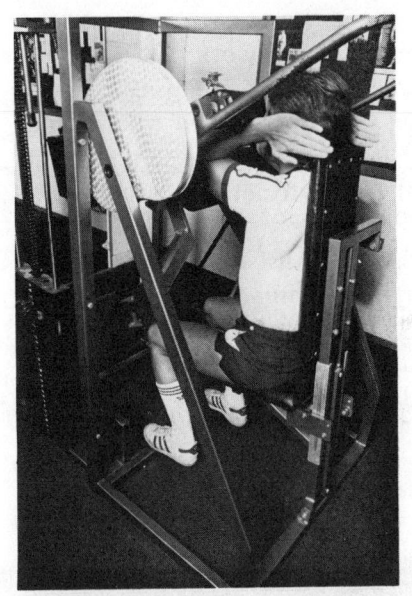

Strength Exercises 93

The Nautilus triceps press.

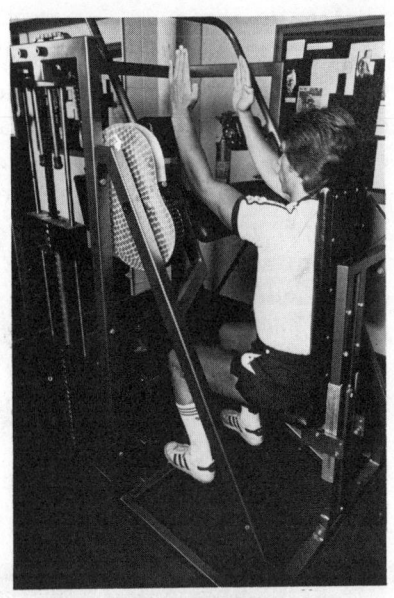

Arms rest on the top of both pads.

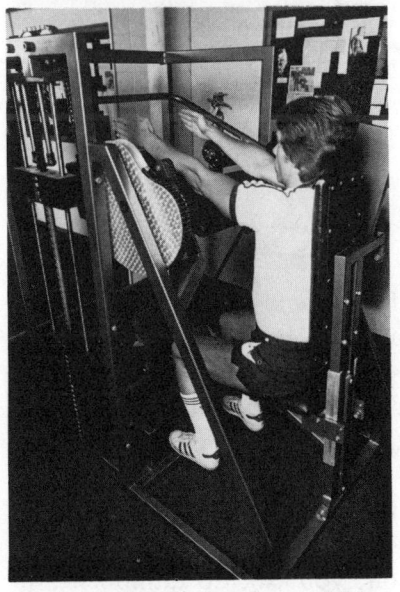

Nautilus machines isolate the muscles.

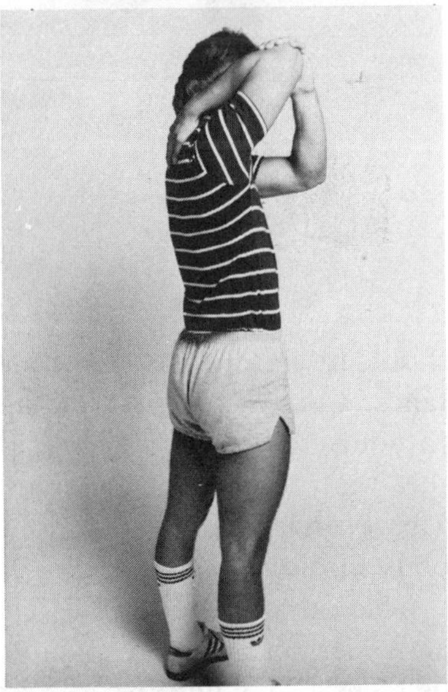

Your bent arm should pass behind your head.

5b Arm flexion

Arm flexion is accomplished largely by the work of three muscles: biceps, brachioradialis, and brachialis. The biceps is the muscle on the front of the upper arms, that is displayed when someone says, "Show me your muscle." It attaches to the shoulder and the lower arm; the two muscles of less notoriety are attached to the upper and lower arm bones.

There are three types of exercises for the arm flexors: rows, curls, and chinups. Rows and curls are similar exercises, except that the grip is reversed.

There are many variations to arm curls but all use an underhand grip. At a standing position hold the barbell with your hands

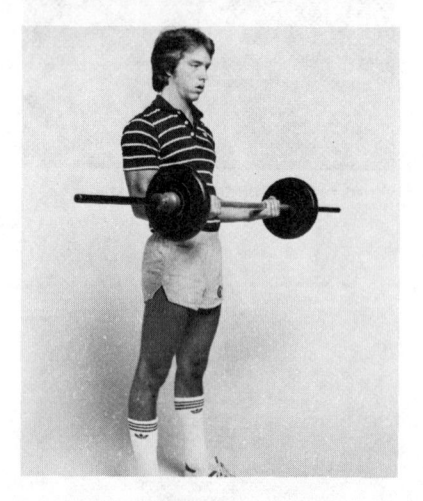

Do arm curls with an underhand grip.

shoulder-width apart. Keep your feet spread about the same distance. Curl your wrists and arms upward, bringing the barbell up to your chest as you exhale; then, lower the weights slowly. Make sure that you do not rock back and forth while doing the exercise. This exercise can also be done while seated; this eliminates some body motion.

This same exercise is often done with dumbbells, again using an underhand grip. Arm motion is alternated when doing dumbbell curls. To improve the isolation, you can do dumbbell arm curls, one arm at a time, over an inclined bench. Rest your arm over the top of the bench and curl the dumbbell upward.

Arm curls concentrate work on the biceps, the brachioradialis and the flexors of the wrist. The wrist muscles are used because they must oppose the forces pulling them downward or extending them.

By reversing the grip from that of the barbell curl and by moving the hands closer together, you do the upright row. In doing upright rows the force of the exercise is in line with the forearms, not

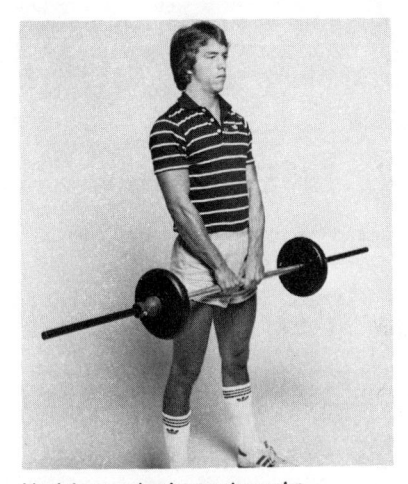

Upright row begins at the waist.

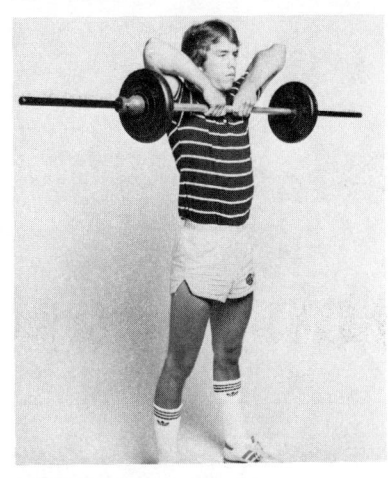

Lift to the chin.

perpendicular to the forearms as it is for curls. Thus, the wrist muscles do little work in rowing. However, rows involve several other muscles that raise the arms. This exercise will be discussed in Section 7, on vertical movements of the upper arm. Bent rows are discussed with exercise Group 6.

Chinnups are a great exercise for the arm flexors. Grab a high bar with an underhand grip, with your hands shoulder-width apart. From a free-hanging position, pull yourself up until your chin is even with the bar and then lower yourself to the hanging position. Do not swing back and forth or kick your feet to help accelerate yourself upward. As you widen the grip in chinups, you involve the latissimus dorsi muscles of the back, which pull the upper arms down. Wide-grip chinups are recommended for this muscle group.

Chinups are difficult for many people. An easier version, called partial chinups, uses a low bar instead of a high one. The bar should be at about chest height or lower. Position yourself under the bar and grasp it with an overhand grip, shoulder-width apart. Place your feet far enough in front of the bar so that you get a good amount of weight on your arms. Pivoting about your heels, pull yourself upward until your chin touches the bar. If you have several bars at different heights, you can vary the exercise difficulty as desired.

For a biceps (and the chest muscles) stretch, stand near a doorway or post. Grasp the post with one hand. Twist your body away

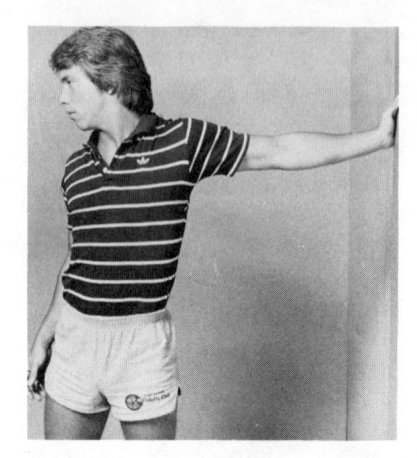

Extend your arm to stretch the bicep.

from the arm so that it is fully extended at the elbow. Continue to turn until you find a comfortable stretch.

GROUP 6: HORIZONTAL MOTIONS OF THE UPPER ARM

It is common to find half of the Group 6 motions unrepresented in exercise programs and the other half represented as arm extension exercises. The muscles that pull the arms together across the chest, the adductors or pectorals, are usually included in exercise programs only at the bench press. The opposing muscle groups, which abduct the arms, are often left out entirely. This oversight creates a muscle imbalance, which results in forward-drooping shoulders and ill-fitting clothes.

6a Abductors of the arms

These are the exercises that are overlooked in strength building programs. To prevent a muscle imbalance and resulting poor posture, balance strong adductors with strong abductors.

There are several muscles that contribute to abduction. Some attach to the shoulder blades and pull them together (shoulder blade adduction), which abducts the arms. The largest of these muscles is the trapezius, a triangular-shaped muscle that covers much of the upper back. The rhomboids, which lie beneath the trapezius, also pull the shoulder blades toward the spine. Latissimus dorsi, teres major and teres minor attach to the upper arm and pull it back and toward the spine. Horizontal motions of the upper arm and shoulder, thus, require a complex combination of action by various muscle groups. If you do the exercises in this group, all of these muscles will get a workout.

One of the best exercises is the bent row. Rowing exercises were mentioned in Group 5b along with arm curls. Rows use an overhand grip. For this exercise, separate your hands as far as possible

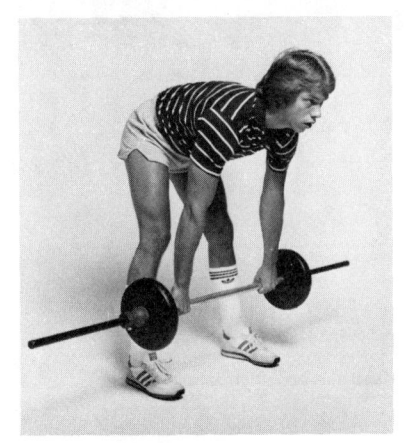

Bent row with barbell.

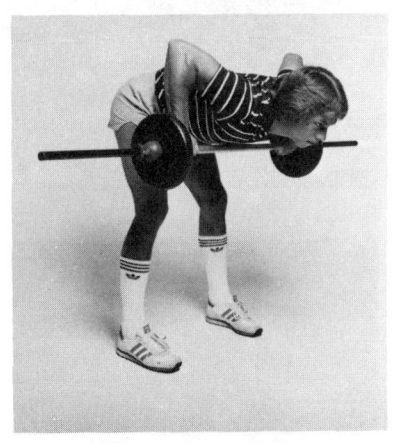

Keep the arms spread.

on a barbell. Starting from a standing position, keep your back bent so that it is horizontal and bend your knees. Raise the bar to your chest and lower it at a controlled rate. Start this exercise with a light weight and gradually increase it. If you have weak lower back muscles, skip this exercise until you have strengthened them. A way to protect your back muscles is to support your head on a bench.

A similar exercise can be done with dumbbells: the alternating dumbbell row. Take the same position as above, with palms facing inward. Alternate raising and lowering the dumbbells.

The last exercise in this group is the bent lateral raise. This is the reverse exercise of the supine lateral flies, and in analogy with that exercise, this one is commonly called reverse flies. Bend at the waist while standing and keep your back and knees bent. Pick up a pair of light dumbbells and hold them so your palms face one another. Then, with elbows held straight, raise the weights out to the side as far as possible.

98 STRENGTH EXERCISES

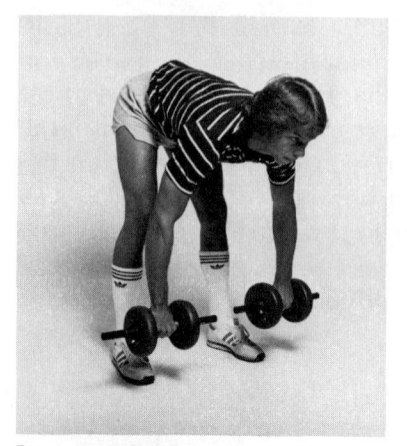

Bent row with dumbbells.

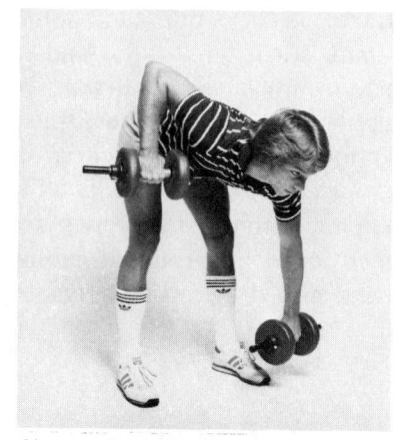

Alternate both arms.

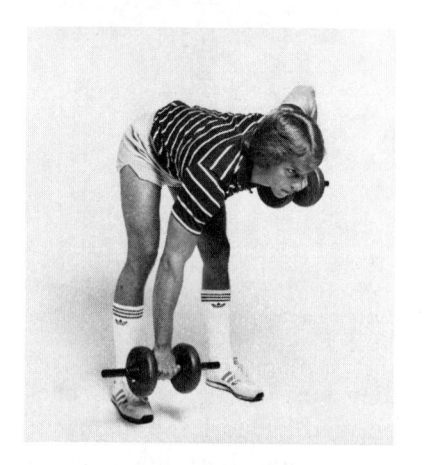

Keep the back bent and steady.

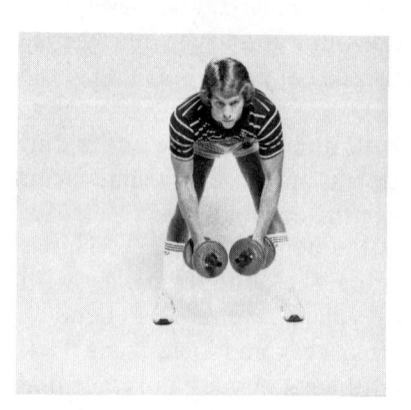

The bent lateral raise.

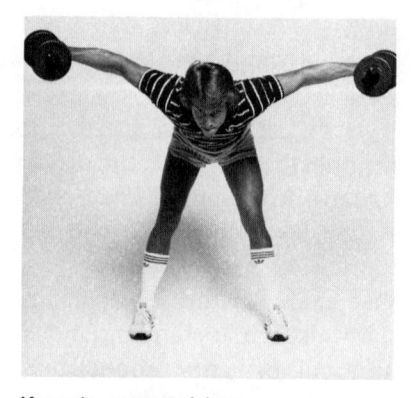

Keep the arms straight.

Strength Exercises 99

The initial motion in reverse flies is almost parallel to the floor while at the later stages it is almost vertical. Thus, the exercise intensity varies greatly. Initially there is little exercise resistance, but when your arms are out to your sides the exercise resistance is at maximum. This causes a tendency to accelerate the weights at the initial angles so that less work is needed when the resistance is higher. To overcome this make sure that you raise the weights at a slow and steady pace. If you want to exercise the muscles at the initial angles, try doing this exercise one arm at a time while lying on your side.

If weights are not available to you, there are two exercises you can do. The first requires a chest expander. This is a set of springs attached to two handles. You pull the springs apart in front of your chest, keeping your elbows locked. Exercise resistance is changed by adding or removing springs from the set. Chest expanders are available at sporting goods stores.

The second exercise requires a partner, but no equipment. Have

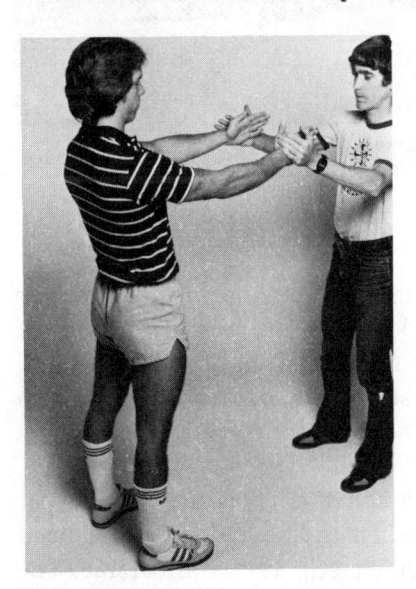

Begin with arms together. 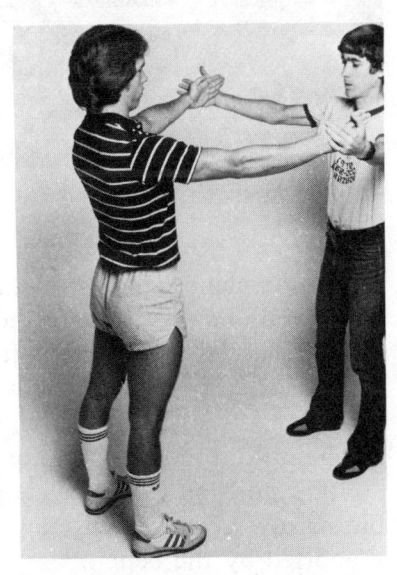   Push against your partner's resistance.

your partner take the place of the springs. He places his hands outside of yours and opposes you as you spread your arms.

To stretch the arm abductors, stand in a doorway or near a vertical post. Grab the post and rotate in, toward your arm.

6b Adductors of the arms

The principal adductors are the pectoral muscles found across the chest. The pectoralis major is attached to the collarbone and sternum and to the upper arm bone near the shoulder. It pulls the arm across in front of the chest. Other assisting muscles are the pectoralis minor, located beneath the pectoralis major, and one part of the deltoid muscles that lies on the front of the shoulder joint.

The most commonly performed exercise for the adductors of the arm is the bench press. A narrow grip version of this exercise

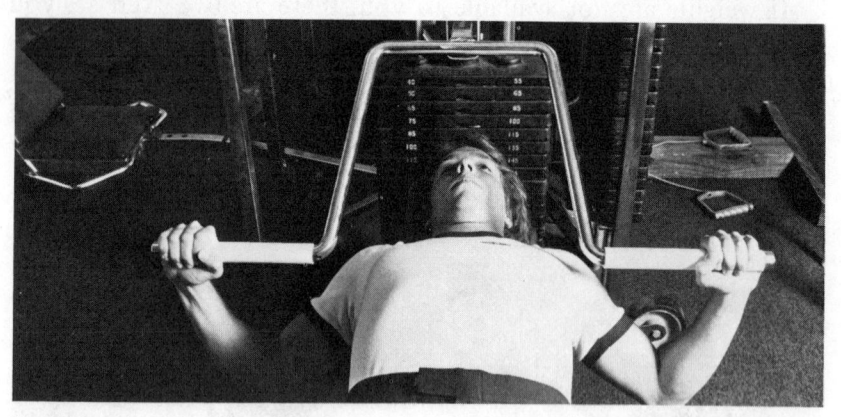

Work the adductors with a wide grip.

was recommended for strengthening the extensors of the lower arm, Group 5a. To exercise the adductors, use a wider grip. Both sets of muscles are involved to some degree, no matter what the hand spacing. Even with the widest grip the exercise requires arm extension as well as adduction, but by varying the grip spacing you emphasize one muscle group or the other.

Body position for the wide grip bench press is the same as for the narrow grip. Lie on your back on the bench with your head supported by the bench. Use as wide a grip as is comfortable. The recommended breathing pattern is to inhale either when your arms are fully extended or while you are flexing them. Exhale while exerting the maximum effort of raising the weights. You will probably find that while using the wider grip spacing you will need to reduce the weight you use for the narrow-grip bench press.

Wide-grip pushups can also be used in this exercise group. Spread your hands wider than shoulder-width. Rotate the position of your hands outward 45°. Then do your pushups.

A second exercise with weights is the supine lateral raise, also called flies. Lie with your back down on a bench. Grasp dumbbells

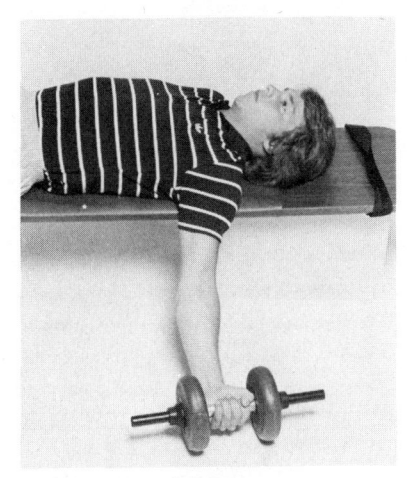

The flies require a bench.

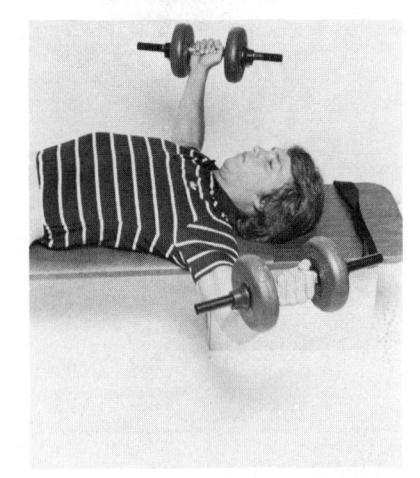

Don't lose control of the weights.

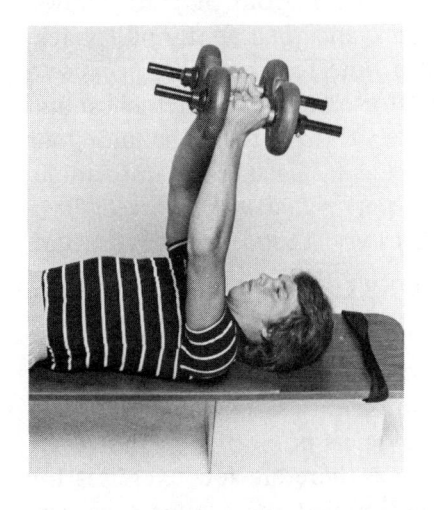

Lift the dumbbells over your head.

on the floor in each hand with your palms facing upward. Bend your elbows slightly and raise the weights directly over your chest. Then lower them to the floor and repeat. The bend in the elbows makes your arm muscles (biceps) work isometrically but relieves stress on the elbow joint.

One of the best stretches for the arm adduction requires a partner. Kneel with your hands behind your head. Have your partner

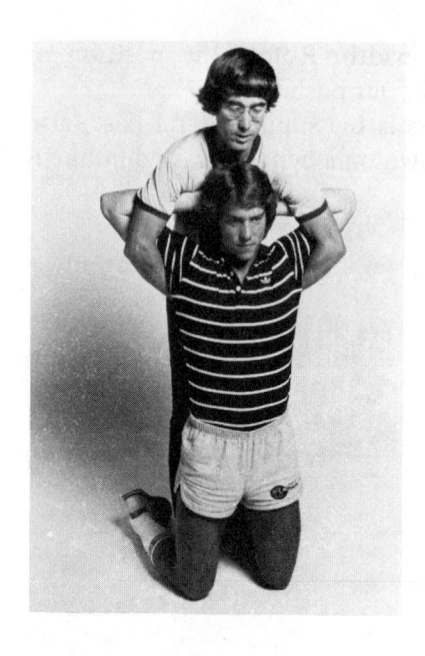

Horseplay is not recommended here.

come up behind you and place his arms in front of your elbows. He clasps his hands behind your back and then gently pulls backward on your elbows. This is not a time for horseplay because a partner can easily hurt the person stretching. To stretch chest and shoulder muscles without a partner, grasp a towel behind your head. Pull it up, over your head and as far back as is comfortable. An entire series of stretches can be performed with a towel. Try a variety of positions to see which gives you a good stretch sensation.

GROUP 7: VERTICAL MOTIONS OF THE UPPER ARM

Included in this group are four motions—raising the arms (vertical abduction), pulling them down (vertical adduction), and elevating and depressing the shoulder. The last two do not really belong in this group from a kinesiological point of view; however, there is overlap in exercises and since there are few exercises for abduction and adduction, we have lumped the groups together.

7a Abduction

The deltoid pulls the arm upward. It is located on the outer or lateral side of the upper part of the upper arm. It is attached to the collarbone and the upper arm bone. There are three parts to the deltoid. The middle part pulls the arm directly out to the side and upward. The front and back parts pull upward plus forward or backward.

To isolate the middle part of the deltoid, do a lateral raise with dumbbells. Use an overhand grip and keep your knuckles pointed directly out to the sides. Starting from a standing position with

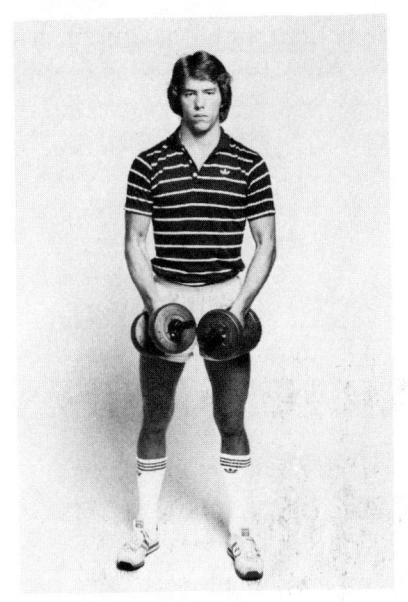

Arm elevators for the deltoids.

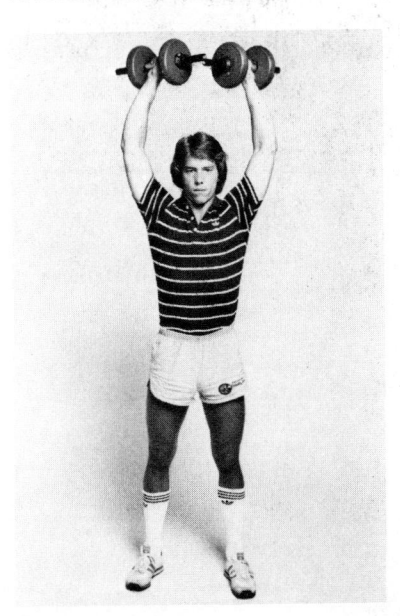

Don't bend the elbows.

Use a manageable weight.

104 STRENGTH EXERCISES

the weights at your sides, raise them up until they are overhead. Lower them at a slow and controlled rate. It is a good practice not to bump the dumbells together over your head—even a gentle bump can fracture the cheap steel in a one-piece dumbbell. I have seen it happen. The Nautilus double-arm machine mimics this deltoid exercise.

To emphasize the front part of the deltoid, hold the dumbbells in front of you instead of out to the side. Use an overhand grip

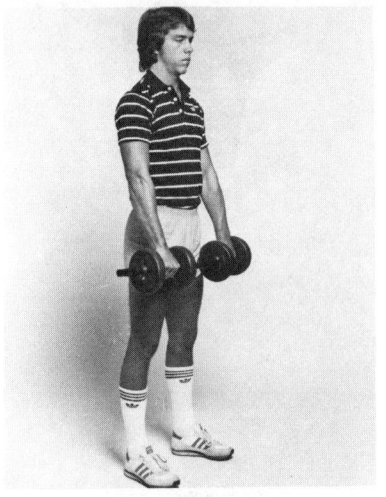

The front raise with dumbbells.

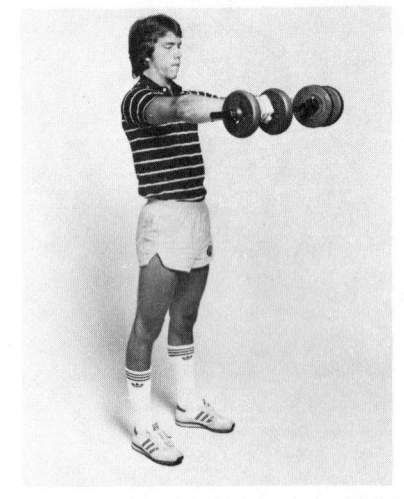

Hold them in front of you.

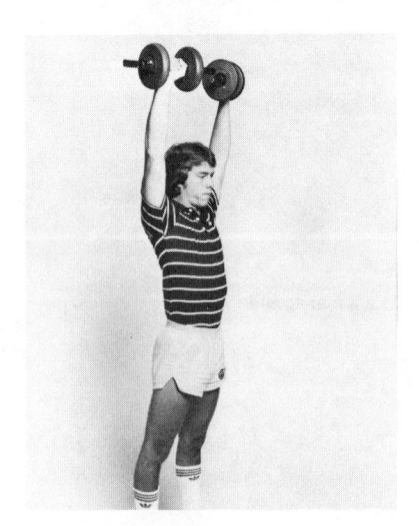

Swing over your head.

and keep your knuckles pointing upward, not out to the sides.

This is a good exercise to do in front of the mirror (as are many others). The mirror allows you to check your exercise form and to see which muscles tense and contract during the exercise.

One of the rowing exercises, the upright row, is beneficial to deltoid development. This exercise involves other muscles, the biceps and parts of the trapezius, but is still very good for deltoids. From a standing position use an overhand grip with your hands close together. Keep your elbows out to the side throughout the exercise. Raise the bar smoothly to your chin and return to the starting position. Do not let the bar fall without resistance—lower the weight, do not drop it.

The last exercise in this group is the military press. It was presented as part of Group 5a, exercises for arm extension. Since this exercise requires that the upper arm be lifted, it is also good for the deltoids. Stand with your feet flat on the floor, shoulder-width

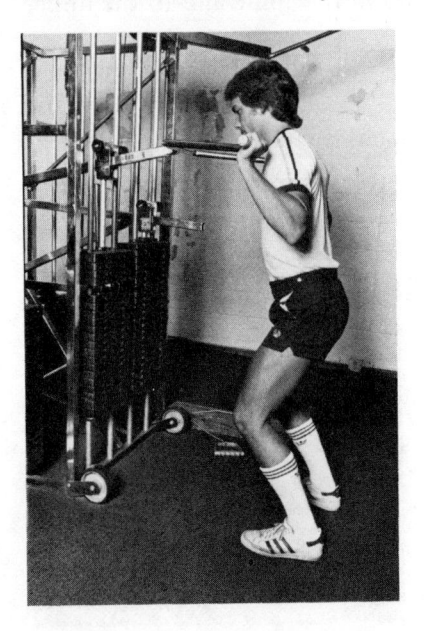

Standing military press moves the upper arms.

apart. From the starting position of holding the bar just beneath your chin, press it upward. Again, watch for extraneous motions of the legs or back that would help accelerate the weights, thus reducing the isolation. This exercise can be done standing with your back to the exercise station. From this position you strengthen the back part of the deltoid.

One of my favorite stretches is at the lat station. (If a lat station is not available, use a fence or other handhold that is about shoulder-high.) Spread your arms and hold onto the bar with an overhand grip. Then let your upper body go limp—supported by your legs and arms. You can move side to side to get stretches for various sets of muscles.

7b Adduction

Adduction, or pulling the arms down, is accomplished by the latissimus dorsi (lats) and teres major, which are located in the back, and by the part of the pectoralis major which attaches to the chest bone and the upper arm. Since exercises for the chest muscles have been given in Group 6b, we will not discuss them here. The lats are a broad set of muscles that cover almost all of the lower back. They attach to bones in the spine and to the upper arm.

The best exercise for this group is the lat pulldown. This exercise requires a lat station, which is available on many exercise machines. Facing away from the machine, hold the bar at the ex-

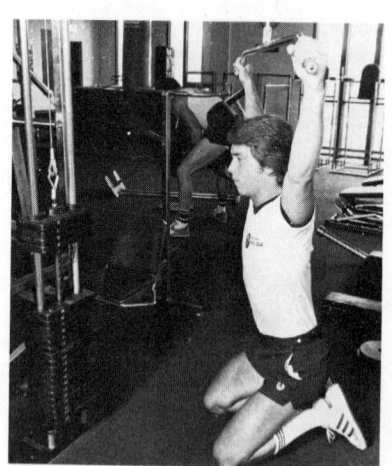

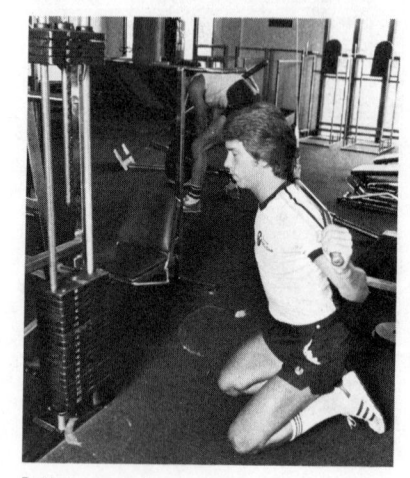

Lat pulldown behind head.

Pull down as far as you can.

treme ends. If you have short arms, you may need to use a more narrow hold. Grip the bar in the overhand fashion. With your arms extended upward, kneel directly below the center of the bar. Now pull the bar down so that it touches the back of your neck. Be careful not to bend your back or hips to help accelerate the weights. If using heavy weights, something approaching your body weight, you will pull yourself off the floor at the start of the exercise. To overcome this, sit with your legs crossed and place one or two 25-pound barbell plates on your lap. If you do not have access to a lat station, rely on wide grip chinups to exercise your lats.

A second exercise at the lat station is the straight-arm pull. Stand facing the machine and grasp the bar with an overhand grip,

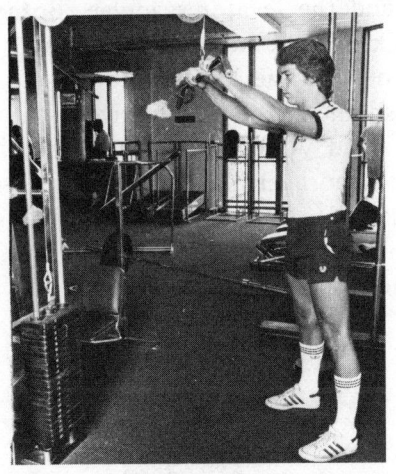

Straight arm pulldown with lat machine.   Keep the arms straight.

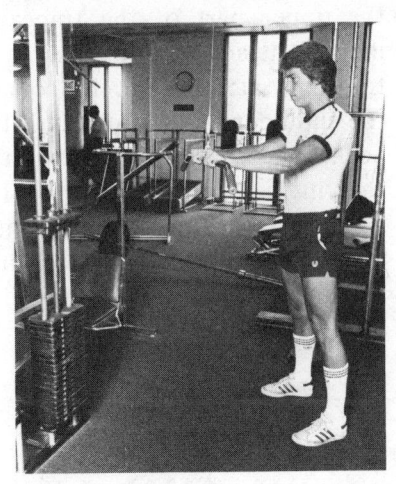

hands about shoulder-width apart. Keeping your arms straight at the elbows, pull the bar down in an arc until the bar is close to your thighs. Then lower the weight (raise your arms) at a slow and controlled rate.

As mentioned earlier, wide-grip chinups are good exercise for the latissimus dorsi. Use an overhand grip at double shoulder-width separation. Pull yourself up to the bar, leaning your head forward so that you touch the back of your neck to the bar.

A simple stretch for the lats and the other vertical adductors is to hang from a high bar. Use a bar that is high enough so that your feet will not touch the ground while you are stretching. Use an overhand grip. Relax all your muscles, except for your grip. If you have a strong grip, try a one-hand hang. From the two-hand position, slowly release the grip on one hand and try hanging from the other hand.

7c Elevation and depression of the shoulder blade

Depression, or downward movement, of the shoulder blade is largely the work of the lowest part of the trapezius. This will get a workout while doing the Group 7b exercises and some of the other arm and shoulder exercises. For this reason, we will not further discuss actions that lower the shoulder blade.

Exercises for raising the shoulder blades, however, have not been given elsewhere. Elevation is caused primarily by the pull of the upper part of the trapezius and the levator scapulae. Both muscles attach to bones in the neck. On the other end, the upper trapezius attaches to the collarbone and the levator attaches to the shoulder blade. Both pull the shoulder upward, relative to the neck. These are the muscles that hold your shoulders up when carrying heavy suitcases across long airport terminals.

To exercise the elevator muscles, do shoulder shrugs with a barbell or dumbbells or at the bench-press station of a weight machine. When using dumbbells, hold them with an overhand grip

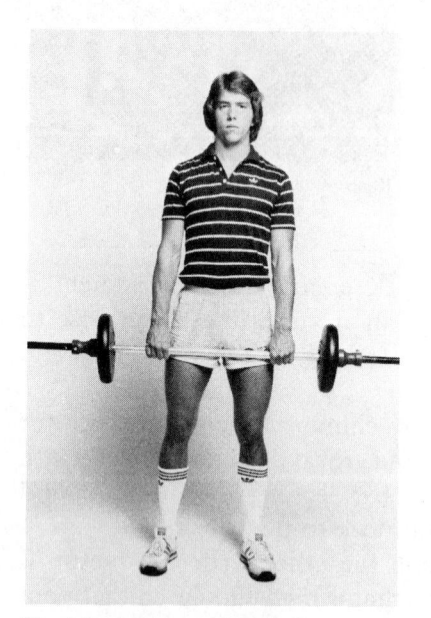

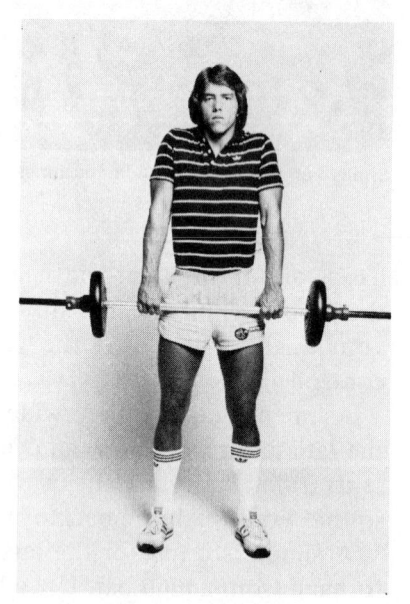

Shoulder elevators with barbell.   These exercise the elevator muscles.

with your arms hanging straight down at your sides. Raise your shoulders either together or alternately. Think of touching your ears with your shoulders. Concentrate on keeping your elbows straight.

Strength Exercises 109

With a barbell, or at the bench-press station, grasp the bar using an overhand grip with your hands shoulder-width apart. Raise the bar to the starting position, which is standing with your legs and back straight holding the bar in front of you. Then pull your shoulders upward.

It is helpful to do this exercise in front of a mirror so that you can watch your form. The most commonly made error is bending the elbows. This allows the arm flexors to assist in raising the weights. If you have not done shoulder shrugs before, you may find the motion awkward. If so, do the exercise for a few sessions with very light, or no weight. As the exercise becomes more comfortable to do, increase the resistance.

Some value for the shoulder elevators can be derived from a variation of the military press. The value is small compared to that derived from doing shoulder shrugs, so we suggest it only if you do not do shrugs. In this exercise the bar is lowered behind the head instead of in front of it. The same grip—shoulder-width apart, overhand grip—is is used as for the military press. Lower the bar until it touches the back of the neck, then push upward.

To stretch the elevators, stand with your back against a wall.

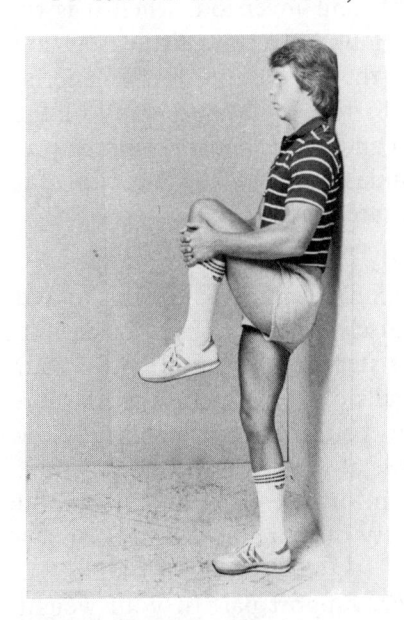

Clasp both hands on the knee.

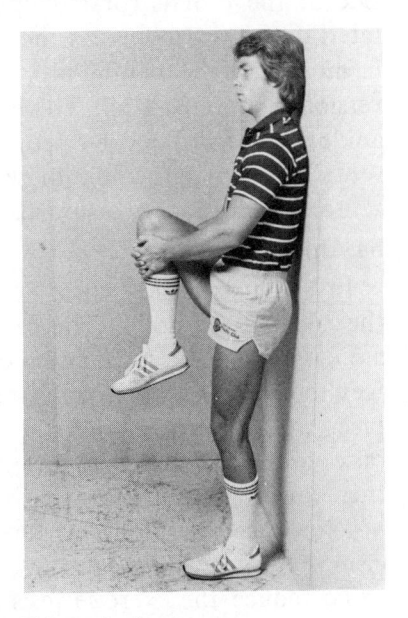

This works the elevators.

Rest your buttocks on the wall. Clasp your fingers together around one knee. With your bent leg pull down on your arms.

GROUP 8: MOTIONS OF THE FOOT

The foot is capable of motion around the ankle joint in two planes. In one plane the foot moves up and down relative to the lower leg. Upward movement by the toes is called dorsi flexion and is controlled by muscles that lie along the front of the lower leg, the region of the shins. Lack of development of these muscles can lead to shinsplints.

The opposing muscle groups lie along the back of the lower leg. These large muscles, including the gastrocnemus and soleus, are commonly called the calf muscles. They attach to the heel by the Achilles tendon, which runs down the back of the leg.

In many athletes the calf muscles are much stronger than those of the shin. This may in part be due to the fact that the calf muscles are easier to exercise. This muscle imbalance, plus the lack of flexibility in the calf muscles, accounts for a large number of injuries sustained by runners.

Motions in the second plane are called eversion, when the outside of the foot is rotated upward, and inversion, when it is rotated downward. Whereas the shin muscles receive little attention in most strength training programs, the muscles of eversion and inversion get none at all. This is unfortunate because many of the ankle sprains suffered by people in and out of sports could be prevented by strengthening these ankle muscles. The muscles that cause eversion and inversion also rotate the foot.

8a Ankle extension

In ankle extension (plantar flexion) the heel is pulled up and the toes moved down. The calf muscles, which cause this action, are easy to exercise. Standing on a step or on a board, move your feet to the rear so that only the balls of your feet are on the surface. Hold onto something to give yourself some stability. Now raise yourself up on your toes. Pause at the upward-most position, then lower yourself down to a comfortable position. Be careful not to exceed the limits of flexibility of these muscles while exercising.

To reduce the exercise resistance, support part of your weight with your hands. To further reduce resistance, do the exercise from a sitting position holding a weight or barbell across your thighs. You can double the exercise resistance of the original calf

Calf raises for the ankles.

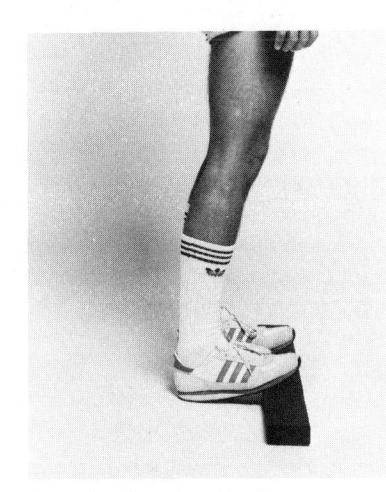

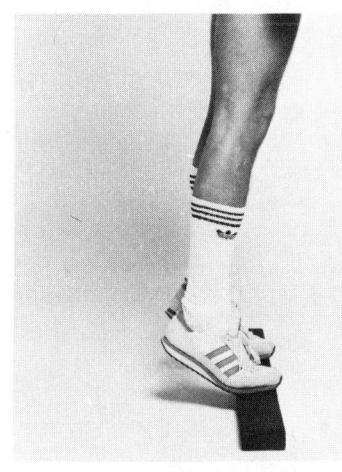

Push off a wood block onto your toes.

raise by doing it one leg at a time. Another way to increase the resistance is to hold a dumbbell in the hand on the same side that the exercise is being done. Use your other hand to stabilize yourself.

A similar exercise can be done at the leg-press station of an exercise machine. Press the pedals forward and hold the weight with straight legs. Now slide your feet down on the pedals so the balls of your feet are supporting the weights. Flex your toes up and down as far as is comfortable.

It is important to carefully stretch both the calf muscles and the Achilles tendon after exercising them. Injuries to the Achilles tendon or to the sheath surrounding the tendon are common because of tightness in the calf muscles. The tightness is caused by strengthening the calf muscle, through running or other exercises, without stretching it, and by the type of shoes worn. Shoes with very high heels allow a shortening of the tendon and muscle, which becomes a problem when shoes are not worn or when shoes with low heels are worn.

The safest way to stretch your calf muscles is to use a wall or a post. Face the wall and place one foot near the wall and the other about two feet back. Put your hands on the wall for support. Keeping the rear leg straight and the front leg bent at the knee, lean forward. You should feel the stretch in the calf area. If not, move the rear leg farther away from the wall. By bending the rear leg and repeating the movement, you stretch the Achilles tendon, which connects the calf muscles to the heel.

112   STRENGTH EXERCISES

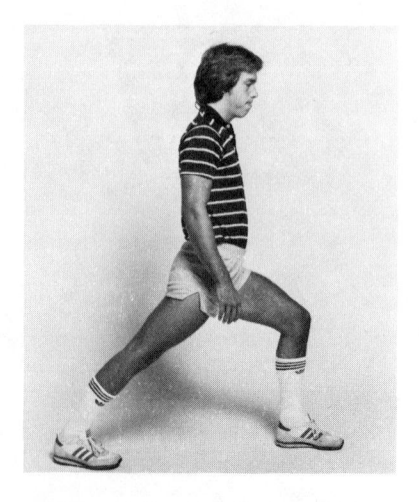

A wall adds stability for the calf stretch.

8b Ankle Flexion (Dorsi flexion)

The dorsi flexion muscles are the weaker members of this opposing muscle pair. Weakness in these muscles, coupled with lack of flexibility, cause or at lease contribute to the majority of the injuries called shinsplints. Unfortunately, few exercise programs include suggestions for these muscles.

To strengthen the muscles that pull the front of the foot upward, you must do the same motion with resistance added. There are two ways to add the resistance. The first is to use an ankle weight (such as a paint can) or iron boot. Fasten an ankle weight around the ball of one foot. Put the heel of that foot on the edge

Try a paint can to work dorsi flexion muscles.

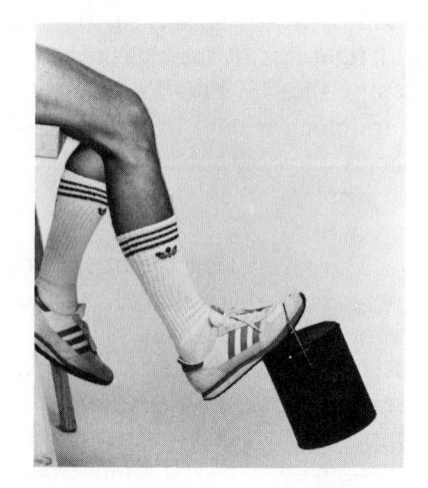

of a step or board so that the foot can be freely flexed upward and downward. Then raise and lower the weight.

The second method requires a partner. Sit on the floor with your legs out straight in front of you. Have your partner place the

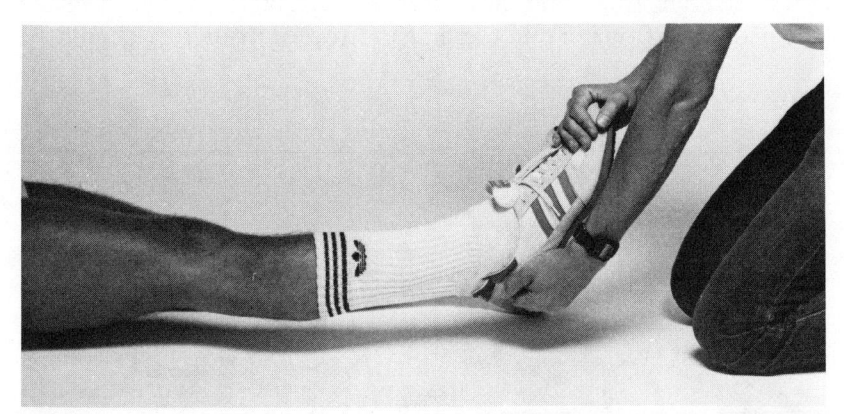

Ankle pull with partner.

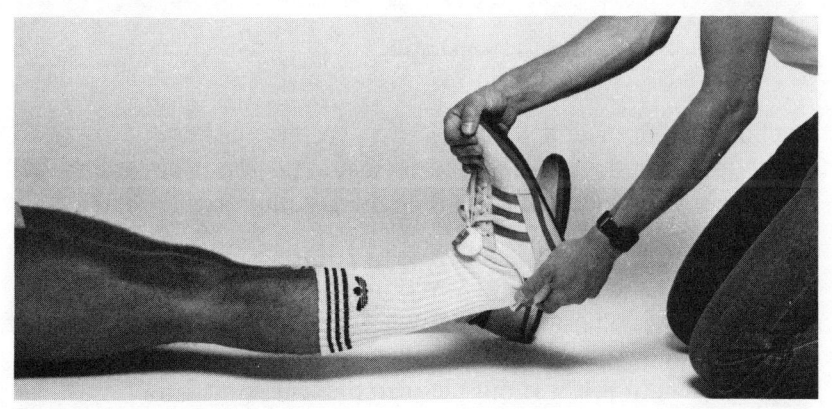

Grasp the foot with both hands.

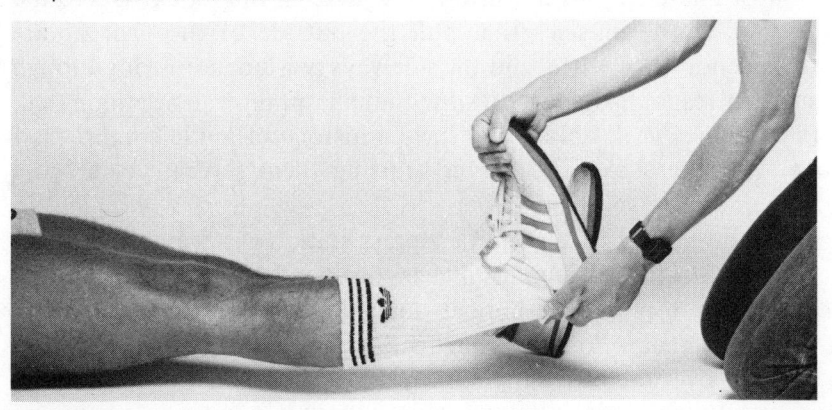

Resist flexion.

palm of one hand over the toes of one of your feet and his other hand cupped beneath the heel of the foot. Then pull your toes upward against his resistance. To start, a light resistance will suffice. Try to do at least 15 repetitions with each foot.

To stretch these muscles after exercising them, lie stomach down on the floor. Your toe and the top of your feet should be

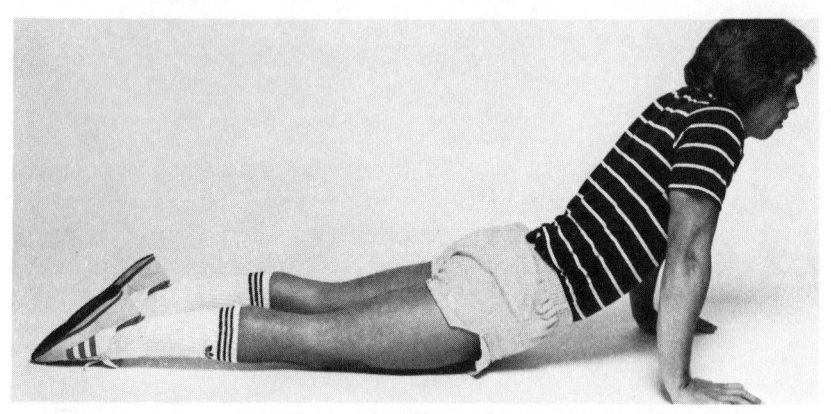

Do pushups with pointed toes to work ankle.

touching the floor and pointing away from your body. Slowly do a pushup and hold the full-arm extension position. To stretch farther, allow your hips to fall, thus arching your back.

8c Eversion

Eversion is the motion of the outside of the foot rising and the inside lowering. The muscles that perform this motion are located on the outward side of the lower leg. They are especially important because strength in these muscles can prevent ankle sprains.

Most ankle sprains are inversions—that is, the foot twists to the outside. If the muscles that pull the outside of the foot up are strong enough to withstand the sideways twist, or are strong enough and can respond quickly to slow the fall, sprains can be eliminated. If you have weak ankles and have a history of ankle sprains (as I do), try these exercises—since starting them several years ago I have not had a sprained ankle.

Stand in front of the military-press station of a weight machine, or in front of a tall bureau. Place your hands and forearms on the bar or on top of the bureau and support some of your body weight on them. Position your feet close together and rotate them outward over the outer edge of each foot. Continue the rotation as far as is comfortable, then return to a regular standing position. Repeat this 15 - 20 times. Support more of your weight with your arms to reduce the resistance. To increase resistance, exercise one ankle at a time with your full body weight. Additional resistance can be supplied by using weights at the military press station.

If you have access to an ankle exercise machine, use it for all of the ankle exercises. Physical therapy departments in hospitals often have the machines. The machines consist of a metal shoe to which you strap your foot. The show can rotate in either the flexion-extension or eversion-inversion planes. If you suffered a sprained ankle, working out on one of these machines will both speed your recovery and help prevent future injuries.

There is another exercise for the eversion muscles. Lie on the floor on your back with your legs straight in front of you. Have your partner place the palm of one hand on the outside of your

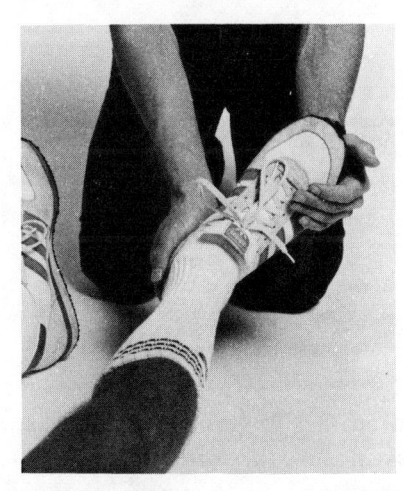

Push against your partner's resistance.

foot. His other hand goes under your heel to keep it from sliding on the floor. You rotate your toes to the outside while he resists. At the farthest point of contraction, he uses more strength, overcoming your efforts, to push your toes to the inside. Then he decreases his resistance just enough so that you can rotate your toes to the outside. Do as many of these ankle rotations as you can.

A similar exercise can be done using rubber or elastic bands for resistance instead of using a partner. Cut strips from a bicycle innertube and tie the ends to make bands big enough so that both feet can fit inside when the band is not stretched. Assume the sitting position described above, with your heels together and with

116 STRENGTH EXERCISES

the band around your feet just below the toes. Rotate both feet to the outside keeping your heels in place. Do 15 - 20 of these. Use wider strips of rubber to increase resistance.

8d Inversion

The mechanics of walking and running dictate that the eversion muscles are the ones that need strengthening more than the inversion muscles. However, to maintain muscle balance, both sets of muscles should get some exercise.

Assume a position similar to the one described above for the partner-assisted exercise. This time the partner places one hand on the inside of your foot. His other hand supports and stabilizes

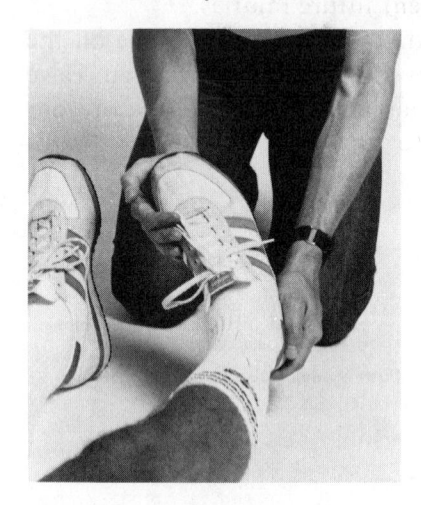

Push your foot inward against your partner's resistance.

your heel. Rotate your toes inward against his resistance and, as before, have him push your foot back in the other direction.

GROUP 9: MOTIONS OF THE WRIST AND HAND

Motions of the wrist and hand are controlled by 25 muscles or muscle groups. Strength in these muscles is very important in racket sports. The same muscles that extend and flex the wrist also rotate it and assist in opening and clasping fingers into a fist.

A simple pair of stretches will reduce muscle soreness and tightness in the muscles that move the wrist and hand. First, stand near a wall and place your hands flat on the wall about chest-high, with fingers pointing upward. Then lean forward. To increase the stretch, move your hands farther down the wall. To stretch the muscles on the other side, form a fist and pull it inward with your other hand.

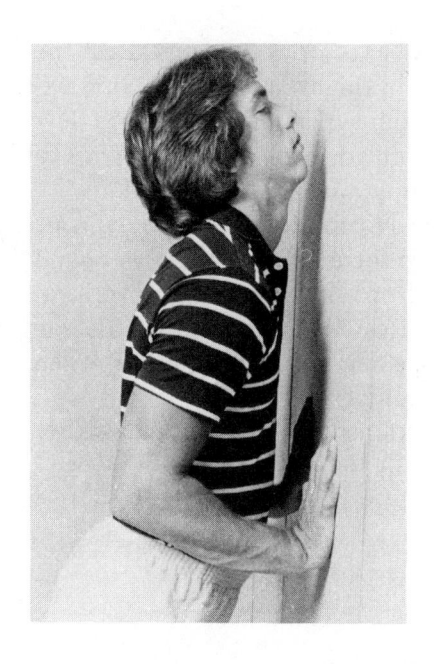

Keep the fingers outstretched and hands as low as possible.

Apply tension on one knuckle, and then another, to accentuate the stretch in different muscles.

9a Extension of the wrist

These muscles attach to bones of either the upper arm or forearm and to bones in the back of the hand. Their action extends the back of the hand upward and back toward the forearm.

Reverse wrist curls are good for developing the extensors. Sit on a chair or bench. Using an overhand grip, shoulder-width apart,

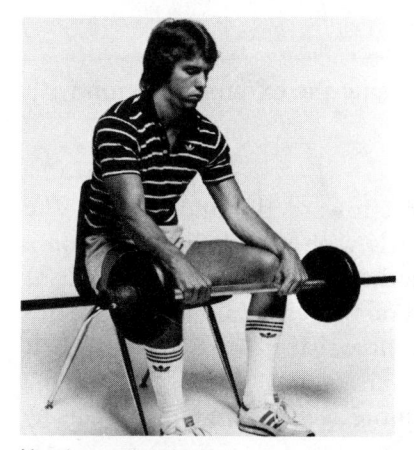

Use the overhand grip.

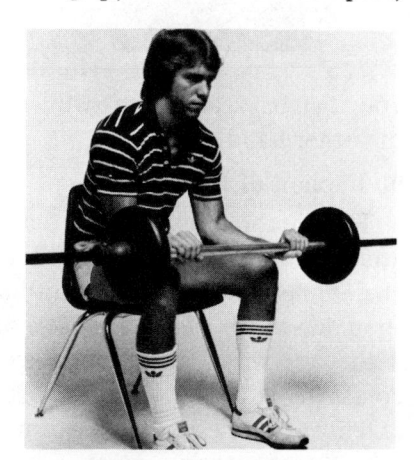

Reverse wrist curls work the extensors.

grasp a barbell with either light weights or no weights. Rest the underside of your forearms on your thighs with your wrists extending beyond your knees. Flex your wrists down as far as they will go and then up as far as they will go. Watch your forearms to ensure that they are not moving during the exercise.

A second exercise is the reverse-wrist rollup. Tie a piece of rope through a half-inch dowel and attach the other end to a five-pound barbell weight. Hold the dowel in front of you with an overhand grip and with your arms straight. Roll the weight up by flexing one wrist at a time, making the rope curl around the dowel. When this has become easy, increase the weight.

To do an exercise for the wrist extensors without using weights, oppose the motion of one hand with the other. Make a fist with the wrist to be exercised. Cup your other hand over it. Then flex

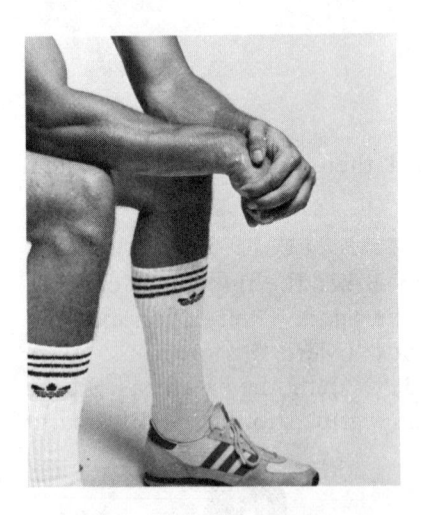

Oppose the motion of your wrist.

your fist back and forth while opposing the extensor motion with the other hand.

9b Flexion of the wrist

The flexor muscles pull the wrist toward the underside of the arm. To exercise them do wrist curls with a barbell. Sitting on a chair, grasp a barbell with an underhand grip with your hands at shoulder-width. Rest the back of your forearm along your thighs with your wrists extended. Flex your wrists down and up to their comfortable limits. These muscles are usually stronger than the extensor muscles, so you can use more weight. To start, try using

Strength Exercises 119

Wrist curl with barbell.

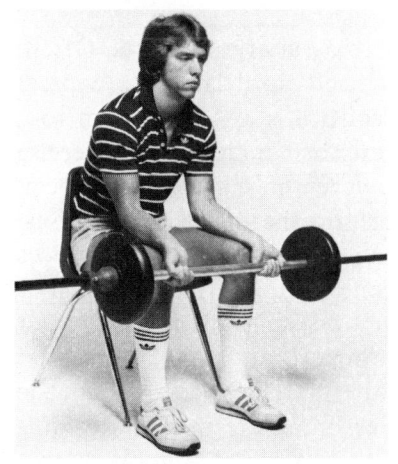

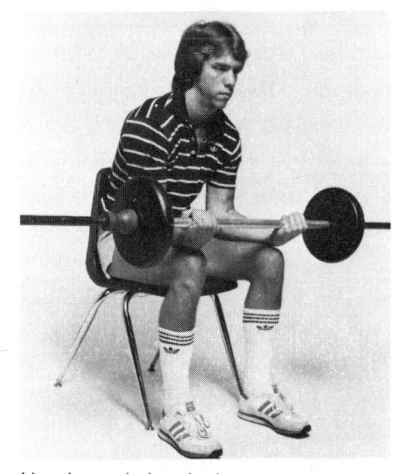

Use the underhand grip.

two five-pound weights on a barbell for wrist curls and no weights for reverse curls.

You can do wrist rollup exercises for the flexor muscles. Repeat the rollup exercise described in 9a, but use an underhand grip.

The exercise without weights is similar to that described above for the extensors. Make a fist and cup the fingers of the other hand

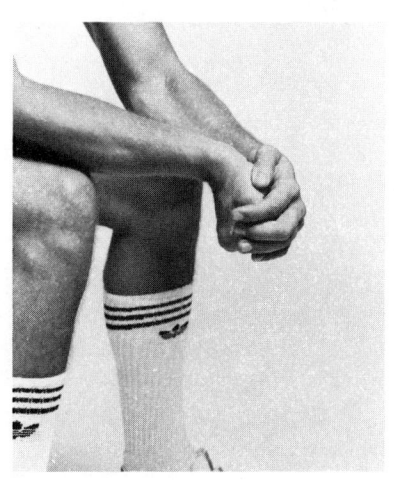

Wrist rollup with underhand grip.

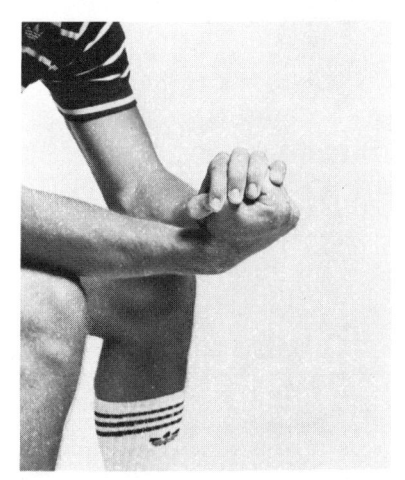

Resist the wrist pulling toward you.

around the fist. Flex the wrist while opposing the motion with the cupped hand.

9c Grip

The strength of grip is important to a variety of sports. Often, lack of strength does not manifest itself until late in a contest when the muscles have tired. Then control is lost and, often too, the game. Many of the exercises described under other exercise groups will build grip strength; however, if you want to specifically improve your gripping muscles, do the following exercises.

Most sporting goods stores have one or more mechanical devices for building grip. If you purchase one of these, make sure it is stiff enough — that is, it has sufficient resistance to overload your muscles. If you can do 20 or more repetitions in the store, it is doubtful that you are overloading the muscles. Use an isometric hand gripper, a piece of hard rubber or plastic molded to fit a hand, to improve your isometric grip for a racket. Choose a gripper, or make one yourself, that is as close to the size of your racket as possible.

A simple exercise is to wad a sheet of newspaper. Place one

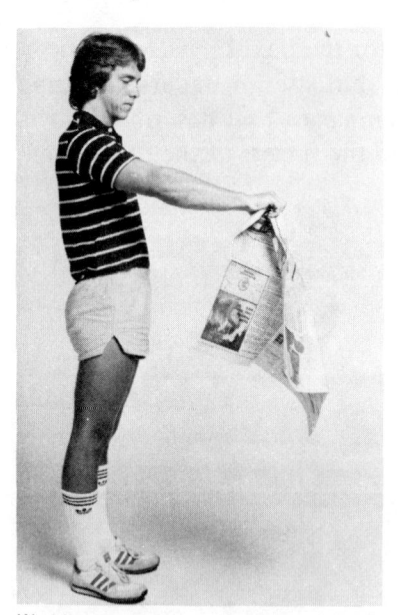

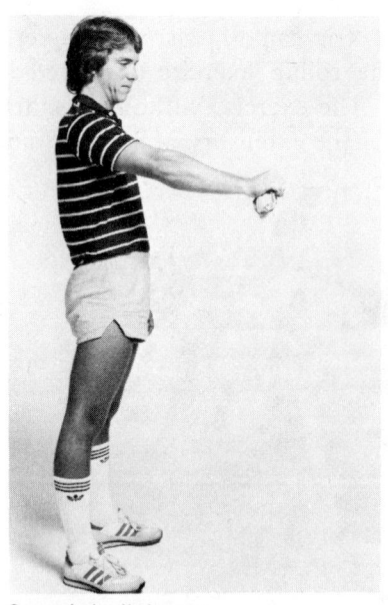

Wadding newspaper works the wrist.   Crumple it all the way.

corner of a full page in your grip. Without assistance from the other hand, wad up the entire page.

If you exercise the grip, you should exercise the muscles that open your hand. Make a fist with one hand and place the palm of

Strength Exercises

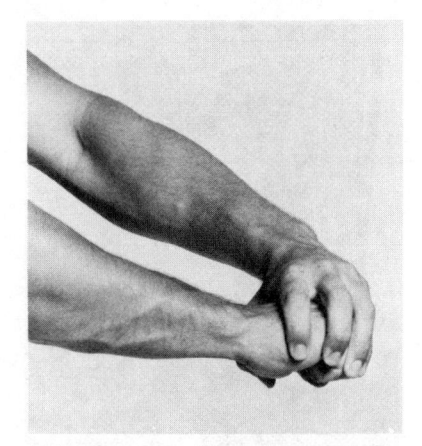

Make a fist, then place palm of other hand over clenched fingers.

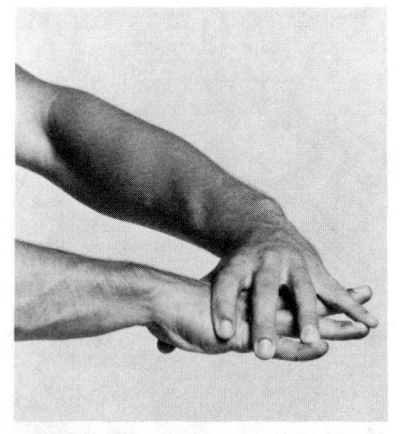

Resist the opening of one hand with the other.

the other hand over the clenched fingers. Open the fist to full finger extension while opposing this action with the other hand.

GROUP 10: MOTIONS OF THE HEAD

Toning the muscles that move the head is important for the prevention of injuries in sports. This is especially true for contact or collision sports.

Using weights for neck extension and flexion requires a special piece of equipment, the head harness or a neck machine. The harness wraps around the head and attaches to a barbell weight by a short strap. Head harnesses are not available at many facilities, so alternate exercises are included here. Nautilus has a 4-way neck machine that is very good for the neck muscles. Use only one plate on the neck machine, to start.

To get a good stretch roll your neck. Start by holding it backward as far as is comfortable and then slowly rotate to one side. When it is tilted forward, hold it in that stretched position and then continue. After a few slow rotations, reverse directions.

10a Extension of the neck

Attach the lead harness to a 2.5- or 5-pound barbell weight. Stand with your feet a little closer than shoulder-width, with your knees flexed. Bend forward at the waist and place your hands on your thighs for support. With the harness wrapped around your head, pull the weight up as far as possible and lower it until your neck is horizontal.

122 STRENGTH EXERCISES

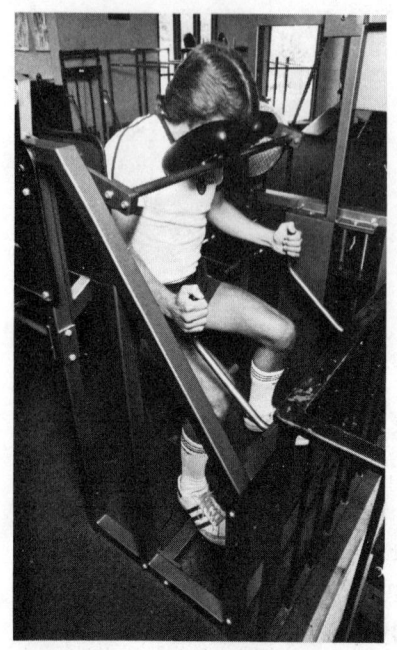

Nautilus 4-way neck machine.

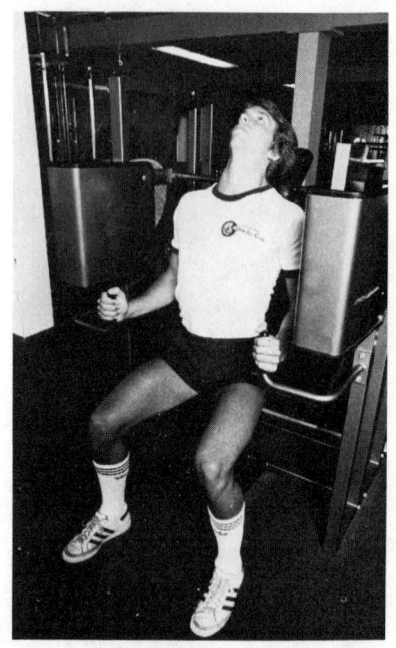

Work all sides of the neck.

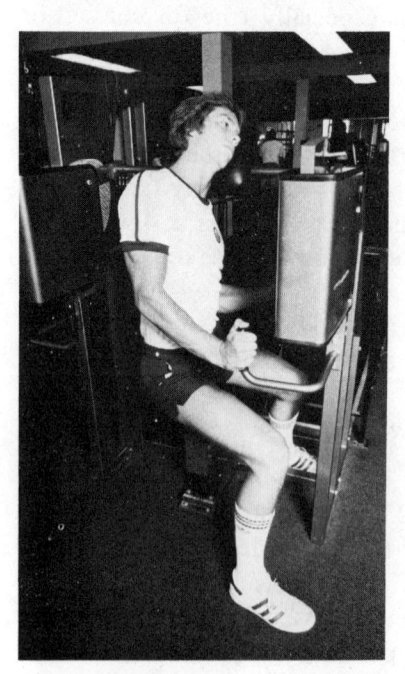

Keep the neck steady.

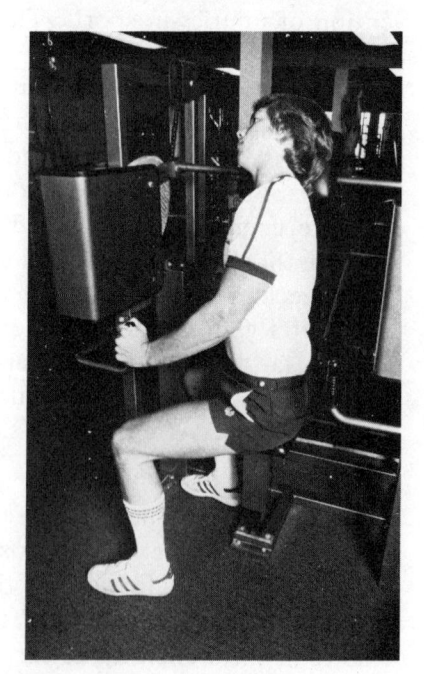

Begin with little resistance.

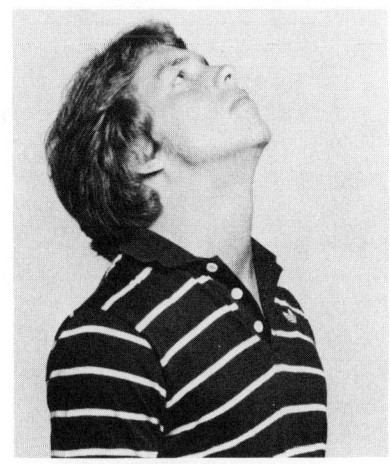

A stretching routine.

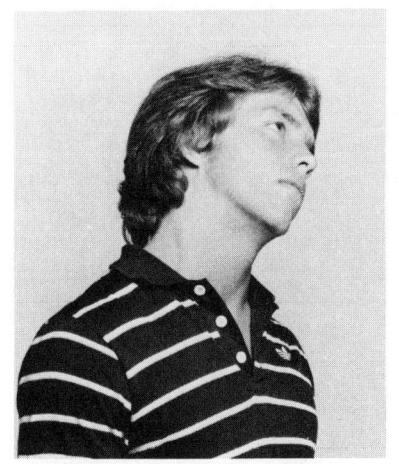

Roll the neck slowly.

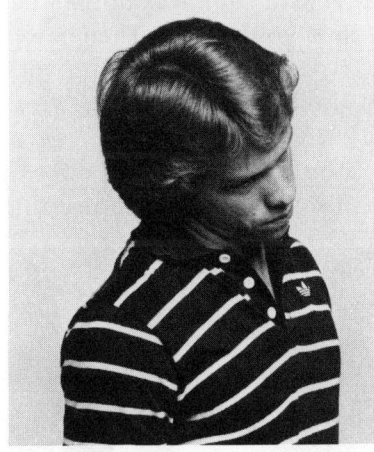

Go to both sides.

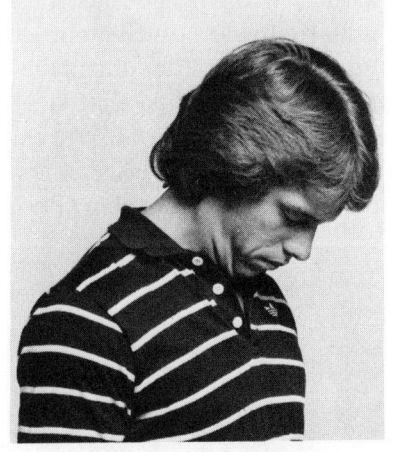

And stretch forward and backward.

An exercise that requires no weight equipment is the neck pull-down. Interlock your fingers behind your head — like you were going to do situps. Pull your head forward with your hands while opposing this motion with your neck. Pull your head down until your chin touches your chest and then let your neck muscles pull your head back up again. Do this initially with light resistance from your hands, and do 5 - 10 repetitions. Gradually increase both the repetitions and the resistance.

10b Neck Flexion

To exercise the flexor muscles, reverse the above two exercises. Using the head harness, lie on your back on a bench. Extend your

124 STRENGTH EXERCISES

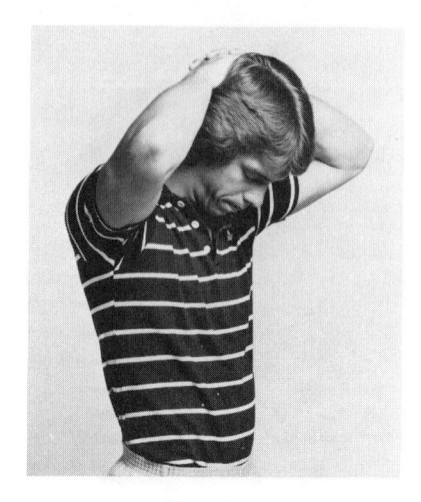

Neck pulldown with locked fingers.

head and neck beyond the edge of the bench and attach the head harness with five pounds or less. Starting with your neck horizontal, pull it upward until your chin touches your chest. Then lower your head to the starting position. Be careful not to overwork these muscles when first starting out. Build them gradually to ensure that you do not injure them.

The second exercise is the head pushup. Place the palms of both hands beneath the chin. Push up with your hands while resisting

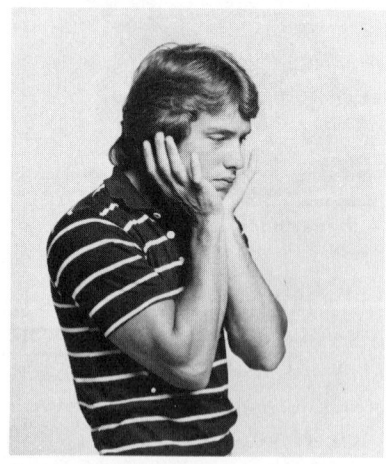

Push with your hands against the chin.

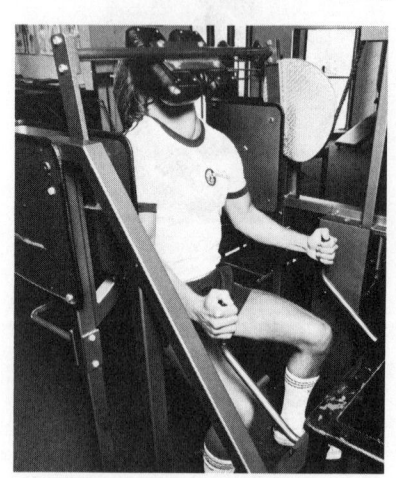

A Nautilus 4-way neck pushup.

with your neck flexors. When your head is as far to the rear as is comfortable, reduce the force of your arms and move your head forward and down. Again, start your exercise program by doing 5 - 10 repetitions with light resistance.

6

Strength Programs for Sports

"A weight-training program for development of strength, power and muscular endurance is one aspect of an allround physical-training program that prepares the athlete for the highly specialized training to follow."

—John Jesse

Athletes and sports people can benefit from strength training in four areas. First, in many activities increased strength can directly lead to improved performance. While this has been widely recognized for athletes in strength sports (for example, in football or throwing the discus or shot) it is only now becoming recognized in other sports. Even in endurance activities, such as running or cycling, strength training is being used to improve performance. For a muscle to endure repetitive contractions it must be strong — but not necessarily large. In sports that require a combination of strength and agility, a lack of strength inhibits improvement. This is often the case for women who may have developed excellent skills but have not tried strength-training programs.

Second, as discussed in Chapter 8, strength training is used to prevent or rehabilitate injuries. The benefits of weightlifting for injury rehabilitation are that the exercise motions can be isolated and can be repeated with the exact resistance that is appropriate for the existing level of strength of each muscle. Also, the injured athlete can use aerobic strength training to improve strength and maintain aerobic fitness while recovering. Strength training is also effective in correcting imbalances between opposing muscle groups, which can result in injuries or poor posture.

Third, strength training is an efficient means of developing the strength needed for a sport or event. Because of the ability to isolate a particular muscle or motion and to work it intensively, strength improvements come quickly. In practicing a sport, some muscles may not be overloaded, thus they will strengthen very slowly. Running can fatigue muscles in the upper body, but running will not effectively strengthen these muscles, because they are not overloaded. If fatigue in these muscles causes poor performance in competition or detracts from training, then a strength-training program would be help an athlete reach his or her potential.

The fourth benefit for an athlete is that he or she can enjoy sports more fully. Achieving one's full strength potential, avoiding muscle fatigue, and staying free of injuries can make a big difference in one's success and enjoyment.

But I must temper the above idea with the idea that the best training for a sport is practicing that sport. Strength training is only one of several tools available to help the athlete. Other tools include stretching, cardiovascular training, and agility drills. Each of these tools can help the athlete in inverse proportion to his existing levels of strength, flexibility, endurance or agility. The weaker someone is, the more improvement that he can gain by strength training. It is interesting to note that the four elements mentioned above are not really independent. Improvements in flexibility can increase the power a muscle produces. Improvements in strength may cause endurance test scores to improve. In one experiment on the agility of children, a group that was given strengthening exercises improved their agility test scores more than those who spent more time practicing their agility test.

The problem with strength training in preparing for a sport is, paradoxically, the same quality that makes strength training so effective — isolation. By isolating a muscle or muscle group it can be overloaded and strengthened; however, improvements in strength will be specific to the angles exercised and a lesser degree to the particular motion and speed of the exercise. Thus, the problem to be overcome is converting strength gained by progressive overloading in restricted motions, to the particular — usually complex — motions of a sport. This is one of the goals of preseason training.

Training for a sport has become a year-round endeavor. Except for a brief rest after the end of the competitive season, the competitive athlete is training continuously. In some sports, practicing the event may not be possible year-round — skiing for example. Strength training, plus training in flexibility, cardiovascular endurance and agility, can be very beneficial in preparing for the season and they can be done anywhere. However, even in sports that can be practiced throughout the year, developing strength prior to starting intensive preseason practice can be beneficial. This is because strength gains come much more quickly in a progressive overload program and these gains can allow the athlete to devote more practice time to refining skills rather than working on strength improvement with inefficient (non-overload) techniques. Once the preseason starts, most of the hours available for training must be devoted to actual practice and few hours are available for strength training; however, the strength gained throughout the offseason can be maintained during the competitive season with only weekly workouts.

I present a generalized seasonal training cycle for all athletes and sports people. When applied to any sport, the length of time spent in each of the training periods will vary, as well as the training regime. Runners will run throughout the year, in season and out; cross-country skiers may use roller skis in the offseason; and downhill skiers may be engaged strictly in strength, flexibility and endurance exercise programs until the snow flies. Realizing that there are these differences to sports preparation, I nonetheless suggest a three-season approach to training.

Offseason training. This may be the longest of the three seasons, depending on your dedication. The goal to be achieved during this time is for improved levels of strength in the muscle groups of particular concern for your sport. You do not gain quality strength in a few weeks of exercising. It takes a firm commitment over your competitive career to develop the strength necessary for championship competition. Start your strength training as early in the offseason as you can.

During this training season you should not be overly concerned with the application of the strength to your sport — that will come later. Concentrate on isolating the desired muscles. Use a lower number of repetitions — no more than 12 to achieve the most efficient strength gains. Start this season doing one set of 6 - 10 exercises and gradually increase the workout to 3 sets.

Mental and physical staleness can be a problem during this period. To help avoid this problem, vary your workouts every 6 - 8 weeks. Change the exercises in your workout. In some cases there will be 12 or 15 exercises in the lists of recommended exercises that follow. Choose 6 - 10 of these and then periodically substitute exercises within an exercise group for muscles that need work, or substitute between exercise groups to concentrate on your weakest areas.

If you are a strength athlete, do the opposite. Decrease the of repetitions performed in each set over the course of the offseason training. Spend the first half of this training period using low repetitions to build strength most efficiently. Develop muscle endurance later in the season. For endurance exercising do 15 - 25 repetitions in each of 2 or 3 sets. Also, you could use an aerobic strength program during the second half of the offseason.

If you are a strength athlete do the opposite. Decrease the number of repetitions during the offseason. The minimum number of repetitions to shoot for is two or three.

Set goals for yourself in terms of the number of repetitions or the exercise resistance. When you meet or exceed your goals reward yourself with a beer or an ice cream cone, or whatever you like. Then set new goals — ones that you can meet in a week or two — and concentrate on meeting them.

Preseason training. Preseason training should take about six weeks. During this time you convert the strength gained in the offseason into improved skill performance in your sport. As skills practice takes up more time there will be less available for strength training. Try to continue strength workouts at least once or twice a week. Their purpose is not to develop more strength — you had the offseason to do that — but to maintain the levels of strength already developed.

Incorporate the exercises that mimic the motions of your sports. These are not recommended for the offseason since they usually do not provide good muscle isolation, which is needed for strength development. But now they are useful. An example of one such exercise is the dumbbell arm swing for runners; this exercise mimics arm swing while running.

Change weights to most closely approximate the conditions in your sport. For endurance sports, use large numbers of repetitions and possibly use aerobic strength training. For strength, athletes use very few repetitions, 2 - 3, but possibly add a fourth set.

Most of your time should now be devoted to practicing your sport. Have confidence that the strength you worked so long and hard to develop will still be available at the end of the competitive season.

Inseason training. If time permits continue strength workouts once a week. Concentrate on those muscles that seem weakest. Your practicing and competition will prevent serious deterioration of strength in the primary muscles used in your sport. Other muscles may show some fatigue and you should exercise them to build up their strength.

PROGRAMS FOR SPORTS

The following pages contain recommendations for strength-training programs for a variety of sports. I have tried to include the more popular sports, but the choices still bear the mark of my own interests.

For each sport there is a list of exercise groups for which an exercise should be done. Where several exercises are listed, choose one of them and use the others as alternatives. I have attempted to keep the number of exercises at a practical limit — around 10. Where I have failed in this attempt, choose 6 to 10, or at most 12, exercises from the list. Pick the ones that will improve your weakest muscles. Vary your workouts by adding exercises from other groups and dropping others.

In many exercises, more than one muscle group is involved, for example the military press. Thus you might find this exercise listed as an arm extensor (triceps) or arm elevator (deltoid). For sports that require strength in both muscles, I have listed the exercise only once.

I have not suggested weights to be used either in terms of pounds or percent of body weight. Start each exercise with a weight you know you can easily handle and perfect your exercise form. Record the weight used and whether you should increase it, decrease it, or not change it for your next workout, depending on the number of repetitions you were able to do. If you were able to do more repetitions than are suggested for an exercise, increase the weight; if you did fewer, decrease the weight. When ready, increase the resistance gradually—usually add 5 pounds for upper-body exercises and 10 pounds for lower-body exercises. Continue to record your weights and reps at each workout to give you a history of your progress.

Remember that in training for a sport you need not have the biggest biceps or thickest quadriceps to win. You must have strength in the primary muscles used in your sport, endurance in those muscles whose fatigue might interfere with your performance, and balance between opposing muscle groups. Use your head in planning a successful strength campaign as much as you use your muscles in carrying it out.

ARCHERY

Competitive archery requires the strength to hold a shooting position without any extraneous motion. Control is essential and control comes through strength development and practice. As in many sports, muscle bulk is not desirable. In fact, recent Olympic gold-medal winners can be described as being skinny—but strong

All of the exercises suggested here are for the wrists, arms and shoulders. If you are shooting, do your strength training after your archery training. I suggest doing 8 - 12 repetitions in each of three sets.

Exercise Group	Motion	Exercises
5a	Arm extension	Pushups, dips, triceps press
5b	Arm flexion	Chinups, curls
6b	Arm abduction	Bent rows, bent lateral raises, reverse flies
7a	Arm elevation	Lateral arm raise, upright rows, military press
7b	Arm depression	Lat pulldown, wide-grip chinup behind the head
9a	Wrist extension	Reverse wrist curls
9b	Wrist flexion	Wrist curls
9c	Grip	Grip exercises

BACKPACKING

Picking up a pack weighing as much as 50 pounds and heading to the hills for a weekend without preparatory exercise is a good way to start a bad weekend. Walking, running and stair climbing are all good exercises. They are even better if you do them wearing a pack with some weights in it. An alternative to wearing your pack everywhere is to do the following exercises. Do these during the dark days of winter and you will find fewer sore muscles on your first few outings. Do 15 - 25 repetitions in 3 sets.

Exercise Group	Motion	Exercises
1a	Leg extension	Squats, leg press, step-ups, leg extension
1b	Leg flexion	Hamstring curls
2a	Hip extension	Swimmer's kick
2b	Hip flexion	Full situps
4a	Trunk extension	Back extension
4b	Trunk flexion	Abdominal curls
7a	Arm elevation	Military press, upright row
7b	Arm depression	Lat pulldown, wide-grip chinups
7c	Shoulder elevation	Shoulder shrugs
8a	Ankle extension	Calf raise
8b	Ankle flexion	Shin strengtheners
8c	Ankle eversion	Ankle roll-overs

BASEBALL

This is an offseason strength-development program. Once practice starts, workouts once or twice a week will maintain muscle strength. Since most of the motions in baseball are explosive, throwing, hitting, or running, your strength program should be, too. Start off by building strength in the 8 - 12 repetition range. Midway through your training program, switch to a power building routine in which you try to do each repetition as fast as possible. Explode on the contraction of each repetition. Do 5 - 8 repetitions and at least 3 sets.

Exercise Group	Motion	Exercises
1a	Leg extension	Squats, leg extension
1b	Leg flexion	Hamstring curls
4b	Trunk flexion	Abdominal curls, side bends
5b	Arm flexion	Dumbbell arm curls, chinups
6b	Arm adduction	Wide-grip bench press

CHART CONTD. NEXT PAGE.

CHART CONTD. FROM PREVIOUS PAGE.

Exercise Group	Motion	Exercises
7a	Arm elevation	Military press, press behind the head; upright rows
7b	Arm depression	Lat pulldown
8c	Ankle eversion	Ankle roll-overs
9a	Wrist extension	Reverse wrist curls
9b	Wrist flexion	Wrist curls
9c	Grip	Isometric grip

BASKETBALL

Basketball requires good leaping ability plus endurance in the leg muscles. It also requires arm strength and endurance—try holding your arms straight up in the air for a few minutes, as if defending your goal. Here is a combination of exercises designed to help strengthen both arms and legs. Do 15-20 repetitions of each in the preseason and 8-12 in the offseason. Aerobic weight training is ideal for basketball players when coupled with a running program.

Exercise Group	Motion	Exercises
1a	Leg extension	Squats, leg extension, leg press
1b	Leg flexion	Hamstring curls
4a	Trunk extension	Back extension
4b	Trunk flexion	Abdominal curls
7a	Arm elevation	Military press, upright row, lateral raises
7b	Arm depression	Lat pulldown
7c	Shoulder elevation	Shoulder shrugs
8a	Ankle extension	Calf raises
8c	Ankle eversion	Ankle roll overs
9a	Wrist extension	Reverse wrist curls
9b	Wrist flexion	Wrist curls

CANOEING AND KAYAKING

The strength requirements of these sports plus the inability for most of us to get out on the water every day, especially in winter, makes strength training essential. Nearly all of the top competitors use some form of strength training. Since these sports encompass a wide variety of events, from pleasure canoeing on a lake, to marathon canoeing, to wildwater kayaking or slalom boating, the following exercises must be integrated into a training program for your specific application.

Aerobic strength training is readily applied to canoeing and kayaking. In fact, I recommend an aerobic strength program geared for specific events. For example, if you are planning on competing in slalom events, which typically last three minutes, set up a circuit training program based on this time. Use a total training time of four minutes. This allows you to do eight exercises: spend 20 seconds at each station and 10 seconds changing stations. Run through a four-minute circuit as hard as you can and then rest for two minutes before repeating it. Do three circuits at a workout. For longer events use longer circuits or eliminate the rest between circuits. Three circuits of eight exercises, with no rest between circuits, will give you 12 minutes of continuous high-intensity training. Add more exercises to make the circuit longer.

I have included exercises for the abductors and adductors of the legs. Choose one or both of these based on the position of your knee braces—usually you use the abductors. The leg press is included to simulate the pressure of your feet on the foot braces. Most of the other exercises are for the arms and shoulders.

For canoeing, where you will be kneeling, add the leg extension and hip extension exercises. One way to work both muscle groups is to use the leg press station facing the other direction. See the photo with the cross-country skiing program.

In the offseason build strength by doing 8 - 12 repetitions. As the season approaches increase the repetition range to 15 - 25.

Exercise Group	Motion	Exercises
1a	Leg extension	Leg press, squats, leg extension
3a	Leg abduction	Lateral leg raise
or		
3b	Leg adduction	Partner-assisted adductor exercise
4a	Trunk extension	Back hyperextension
4b	Trunk flexion	Abdominal curls, situps, side bends
5a	Arm extension	Alternating dumbbell press

CHART CONTD. NEXT PAGE.

CHART CONTD. FROM PREVIOUS PAGE.

Exercise Group	Motion	Exercises
5b	Arm flexion	Arm curls, chinups, dumbbell alternating curls
6b	Arm abduction	Bent rows
7a	Arm elevation	Standing rows, military press, lateral raise with dumbbells
7b	Arm depression	Lat pulldown

CROSS-COUNTRY SKIING

There is still some debate over the value of strength training to cross-country skiing. However, strength training is growing in popularity among competitive skiers and is being recommended more for recreational skiers, especially for the prevention of weekend injuries. Obviously the best training for skiing is skiing. Unfortunately only a lucky few have daily access to good snow. Even those few must wait throughout the summer and fall until conditions favor their sport. Strength training can help prepare the skier for the season and can make the first few outings much more enjoyable—that is, less painful. For competitive skiers, being physically prepared for the start of the season means that they do not waste the first few weeks of the snow season on building strength and endurance.

Most of the training preparation for skiing should be oriented toward cardiovascular and muscular endurance; however, I recommend building strength with low repetitions (8 - 12) during the summer and early fall and then increasing the repetitions up to 30 - 40 and emphasizing endurance as the season approaches. Aerobic weight programs are ideal for ski training.

The exercises recommended here include those for poling as well as for hip and leg action. With the exception of the abductors and adductors of the legs, use up to 40 repetitions on all the exercises during your endurance training. Dr. Art Dickinson, advisor to the U.S. Olympic ski team, recommends doing only strength building exercises, 6 - 10 repetitions, for the abductor and adductors. He reasons that these muscles do not play a direct part in the skiing motion and are needed only for maintaining balance and maneuvering on downhill runs—they do not require high endurance training.

Exercise Group	Motion	Exercises
1a	Leg extension	Leg extension, squats, leg press
1b	Leg flexion	Hamstring curl, one leg lift
2a	Hip extension	Swimmer's kick, leg raise
2b	Hip flexion	Double leg raise, full situps
3a	Leg abduction	Lateral leg raise
3b	Leg adduction	Partner-assisted leg adduction
4a	Trunk extension	Back extension
4b	Trunk flexion	Abdominal curls
5a	Arm extension	Dips, triceps press
6b	Arm abduction	Bent rows, bent lateral raise
7a	Arm elevation	Lateral raises. Do these face down on an inclined board to work the rear portion of the deltoid. Or do military press, pushing the bar up behind your head.
7b	Arm depression	Lat pulldown, straight arm pulldown
8b	Ankle flexion	Shin strengtheners
8c, d	Ankle eversion, inversion	Ankle rolls, ankle rotations inward and outward

Dr. Dickinson recommends other exercises that are more specific to cross-country skiing. For example, in the preseason replace the arm exercises above with two arm swing exercises using dumb-

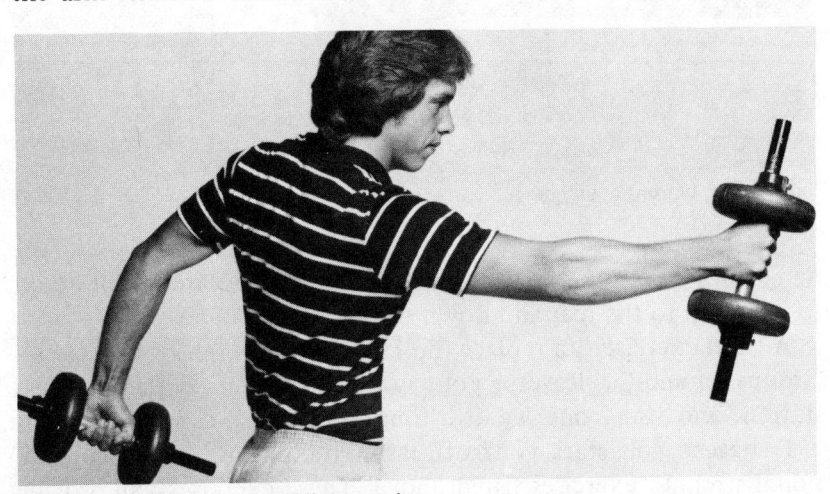

Swinging dumbbells for x-c skiing exercise.

bells. In the first, stand facing a wall and lean toward it so that you are about 30° from the vertical. Spread your feet a comfortable distance and with a dumbbell in one hand swing it backward and forward. Remember that the weight should be heavy enough so that you reach muscle fatigue as you meet your repetition goal of 30 - 40.

The second arm swing exercise is done while you are face down

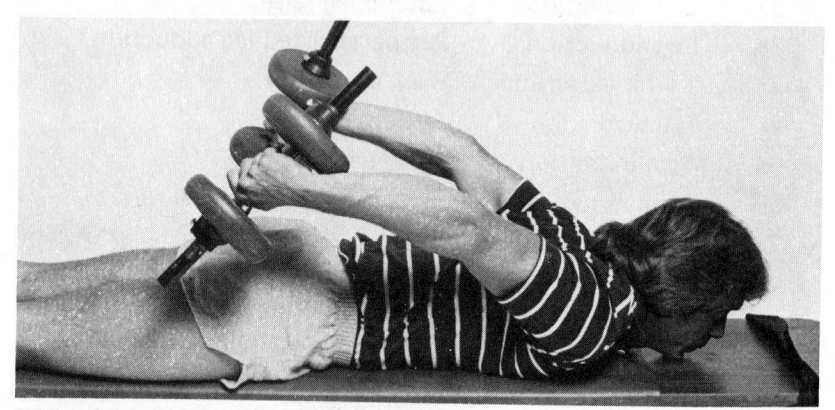

Swing the dumbbells behind your back.

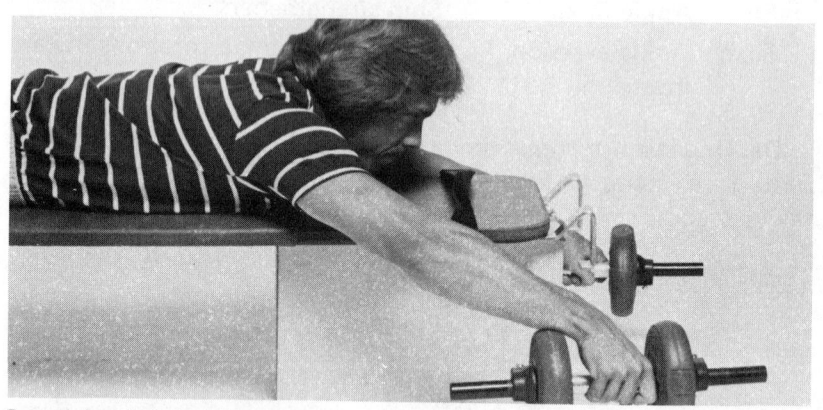

Extend them in front of you next.

lying on a bench. Grab a dumbbell in each hand and swing them together up to the rear and down to the front.

A third exercise can replace the leg and hip extensor exercises—Groups 1a and 2a. Reverse your normal position on the leg press station, and using one leg at a time, push the pedals to the rear.

I suggest you start your offseason training using the conventional strength exercises listed above. These exercises will provide you with more efficient strength gains due to the isolation of the particular muscles. During the preseason, the training objective becomes the application of the newly gained strength to the specific motions of the skiing. At this time switch to the exercises recommended by Dr. Dickinson. Your muscles will maintain their strength since they continue to be exercised, either in the weight room or on the ski trails, and you will also be developing the coordination and specificity of motion that will help you ski better, and, as Dr. Dickinson says, ski funner.

CYCLING

Cycling is another sport in which the value of strength training is gaining acceptance. There are two principal goals of strength training for cyclists. The first is to develop muscle strength and endurance in the prime mover muscle groups in the offseason when weather may prohibit riding. The second is to develop strength in other muscle groups that are not directly involved in the cycling motion, but may fatigue during long rides. Examples of such muscles are the neck extensors, wrists, shoulders, and back.

As with other endurance sports, an offseason strength-development program for cycling should start by using a low number of repetitions, 8 - 12. Just before outdoor training begins, increase the number of repetitions to 30 - 40 to emphasize muscle endurance. As cycling consumes more of the available training time, you can reduce your weight room work. If possible, do a maintenance program once or twice a week. Aerobic strength training is ideally suited for cycling.

OFFSEASON PROGRAM

Exercise Group	Motion	Exercises
1a	Leg extension	Leg press, leg extension, stepups
1b	Leg flexion	Hamstring curls
4a	Trunk extension	Back extension
4b	Trunk flexion	Abdominal curls
5a	Arm extension	Bench press, pushups
6a	Arm abduction	Bent rows
8a	Ankle extension	Calf raises

CHART CONTD. NEXT PAGE.

140 STRENGTH PROGRAMS FOR SPORTS

CHART CONTD. FROM PREVIOUS PAGE.

Exercise Group	Motion	Exercises
8b	Ankle flexion	Toe raises
10a	Neck extension	Partner-assisted extension, 4-way neck machine

PRESEASON PROGRAM

Exercise Group	Motion	Exercises
4a	Trunk extension	Back extension
4b	Trunk flexion	Abdominal curls, situps
5a	Arm extension	Bench press, pushups, dips
6a	Arm abduction	Bent row
7a	Arm elevation	Military press
7b	Arm depression	Lat pulldown
9a	Wrist extension	Reverse wrist curls
9b	Wrist flexion	Wrist curls

DOWNHILL SKIING

Few people have ready access to skiing resorts. When they do get to good snow they should be physically prepared to enjoy the limited time available. Muscles that are taxed by heavy boots and skis soon tire. The more tired the muscles become, the less able they are to correct or recover from mistakes—the chances of injuries then increase.

A fitness program for skiers should include cardiovascular training. The following strengthening exercises can be done in conjunction with that training. Work toward endurance—do 15-20 repetitions at 2 - 3 sets. This program can be continued throughout the ski season. If you are a weekend skier, work out on Tuesdays and Thursdays.

Exercise Group	Motion	Exercises
1a	Leg extension	Squats, leg press, leg extension
1b	Leg flexion	Hamstring curls
2a	Hip extension	Swimmer's kick

CHART CONTD. NEXT PAGE.

Strength Programs for Sports

CHART CONTD. FROM PREVIOUS PAGE.

Exercise Group	Motion	Exercises
2b	Hip flexion	Leg raises
3a	Leg abduction	Lateral leg raise
3b	Leg adduction	Partner-assisted exercise
4a	Trunk extension	Back hyperextension
4b	Trunk flexion	Abdominal curls, situps, side bends
5a	Arm extension	Bench press, pushups, dips
7b	Arm depression	Lat pulldown
8a	Ankle extension	Calf raise
8b	Ankle flexion	Shin strengtheners
8c, d	Ankle eversion, inversion	Inward and outward rotations

FENCING

Fencing is an asymmetric sport in that motions performed with one side of the body are different from those on the other side. One leg always leads, the other always follows. One arm is used only for balance while the other holds and moves the foil. Weight training can be used not only to improve the strength of the muscles used in fencing but also to balance the muscle development in both sides of the body. Use 8 - 12 repetitions for the arm exercises and 15 - 25 repetitions for the others.

Exercise Group	Motion	Exercises
1a	Leg extension	Squats
1b	Leg flexion	Hamstring curls
4a	Trunk extension	Back extension
4b	Trunk flexion	Abdominal curls
5a	Arm extension	Bench press, pushups
5b	Arm flexion	Upright rowing
7a	Arm elevation	Lateral arm raise, forward arm raise (underhand grip)
9a	Wrist extension	Reverse wrist curl
9b	Wrist flexion	Wrist curl
9c	Grip	Isometric grip squeeze

FOOTBALL

Strength training for football has advanced to the point where we cannot do justice to the variety of programs now used. Here is a general program for offseason training for football players. Boyd Epley, strength coach at the University of Nebraska, recommends doing three sets of exercises. In the first, choose the weights so that you can do 10 repetitions. For the second and third sets, aim for 8 and 6 repetitions by increasing the resistance. He also recommends doing all three sets of one exercise before moving on to the next. A 90 - 120 second rest is allowed between sets. For situps, back extension and swimmer's kick do 15 - 20 repetitions.

Exercise Group	Motion	Exercises
1a	Leg extension	Squats, leg extension, leg press
1b	Leg flexion	Hamstring curls
2a	Hip extension	Swimmer's kick, Nautilus hip and back
4a	Trunk extension	Back hyperextension
4b	Trunk flexion	Abdominal curl
5a	Arm extension	Bench press, dips
5b	Arm flexion	Barbell curl
7a	Arm elevation	Military press, upright row
7b	Arm depression	Lat pulldown, wide grip chinups
7c	Shoulder elevation	Shoulder shrug
8a	Ankle extension	Calf raise
8c	Ankle eversion	Ankle roll-overs
10a	Neck extension	Neck pulldowns, 4-way neck machine
10b	Neck flexion	Neck pushups, 4-way neck machine

GOLF

Do 8 - 12 repetitions of the following exercises in 3 sets in the offseason and preseason. Do maintenance exercises at least once a week in the competitive season.

Exercise Group	Motion	Exercises
1a	Leg extension	Leg press, squat
4a	Trunk extension	Back extension
4b	Trunk flexion	Abdominal curls, side bends
5a	Arm extension	Bench press, dips, pushups

CHART CONTD. NEXT PAGE.

CHART CONTD. FROM PREVIOUS PAGE.

5b	Arm flexion	Dumbbell curl, reverse curl, chinups
7a	Arm elevation	Upright row, military press
9a	Wrist extension	Reverse wrist roll up
9b	Wrist flexion	Wrist roll up
9c	Grip	Isometric grip (maximum strength for 6 - 10 seconds, repeated)

GYMNASTICS

Strength is often a limiting factor for gymnasts—this is especially true for young gymnasts. Even minor gains in strength can allow them to make rapid progress. The following program is a general one to be used in the offseason. If muscle weakness is noted in training, strength exercises should be prescribed to overcome it. Do 8 - 12 repetitions in three sets except for abdominal curls or situps, for which you should do 15 - 25 repetitions.

Exercise Group	Motion	Exercises
1a	Leg extension	Squats, leg press
2a	Hip extension	Full situps, leg lifts
4a	Trunk extension	Back hyperextension
4b	Trunk flexion	Abdominal curls, situps
5a	Arm extension	Dumbbell press, dips
5b	Arm flexion	Curl, dumbbell curl
7a	Arm elevation	Upright row, military press
7b	Arm depression	Lat pulldown
8b	Ankle extension	Calf raise

JUDO

Here are some exercises to improve the strength required in judo and other martial arts. Do 8 - 12 repetitions of these exercises in three sets or do them in an aerobic strength workout.

Exercise Group	Motion	Exercises
1a	Leg extension	Squats
2a	Hip extension	Swimmer's kick
2b	Hip flexion	Leg raise
4a	Trunk extension	Back hyperextension
4b	Trunk flexion	Situps, side bends
7a	Arm elevation	Upright row

7b	Arm depression	Lat pulldown
8c	Ankle eversion	Ankle roll overs
9a	Wrist extension	Reverse wrist curls
9b	Wrist flexion	Wrist curls
9c	Grip	Hand grippers
10a	Neck extension	Neck pulldowns, 4-way neck machine
10b	Neck flexion	Neck pushups, 4-way neck machine

MARKSMANSHIP

To shoot consistently, which results in accuracy, throughout a long match requires fatigue-resistant muscles. This is more true for pistol shooters than rifle shooters. Shooting positions for the rifle rely more on support provided directly by bones wheareas positions for the pistol require more muscle support. The following program can help either type of shooter. Do 8 - 12 repetitions of each exercise in three sets.

Exercise Group	Motion	Exercises
4a	Trunk extension	Back extensions
4b	Trunk flexion	Abdominal curls
5a	Arm extension	Bench press, pushups
6a	Arm abduction	Bent rows, reverse flies
7a	Arm elevation	Military press, press behind the head, dumbbell lateral raises
9a	Wrist extension	Reverse wrist curl, wrist roll-up
9b	Wrist flexion	Wrist curl
9c	Grip	Isometric grip exercises

Another exercise for the pistol shooter is to hold a light dumbbell or weight, say five pounds, in the shooting position. Maintain the position for as long as possible. Do several sets of this exercise.

RACKET SPORTS

Although each of the racket sports requires different motions, the strength requirements are similar. The large number of body motions involved in these sports requires a wide range of strength development exercises. For example, a backhand shot uses the trapezius muscles to pull the shoulder blades together. A forehand shot uses the pectoral muscles, the horizontal adductors of the arms. Strong deltoid muscles are needed to hold your arm and racket up, away from your body. Overhead shots and overhead serves bring the arm depressors into play.

From the following list pick the 8 - 10 exercises that will help you the most. For example, if you have been running throughout the offseason, you might skip leg extensions and curls and concentrate more on arm and shoulder exercises. Do 8 - 12 repetitions. To improve your grip strength, do repeated isometric grips on an object the same size as your racket handle. Exert maximum strength for six seconds. Repeat this several times.

Exercise Group	Motion	Exercises
1a	Leg extension	Leg extension, squat
1b	Leg flexion	Hamstring curls
4a	Trunk extension	Back extension
4b	Trunk flexion	Abdominal curls, side bends
5a	Arm extension	Bench press, pushups, dips
5b	Arm flexion	Reverse barbell curl
6a	Arm abduction	Bent lateral raise
6b	Arm adduction	Wide-grip bench press, pushups, flies
7a	Arm elevation	Military press, lateral arm raise
7b	Arm depression	Straight arm pulldown
8b	Ankle extension	Calf raise
8c	Ankle eversion	Ankle rolls
9a	Wrist extension	Reverse wrist curls
9b	Wrist flexion	Wrist curls
9c	Grip	Grip exercises, isometric grip

RUNNING

The benefits of strength training for a runner have been well-documented over the past few years. Some people still dispute the value for competitive, long-distance running; however, more distance runners are now using weights than ever before.

For the competitive runner, strength training can serve four functions. First, it builds power or endurance, depending somewhat on the training methods, in the driving muscles of the legs and hips. Second, it develops strength in muscles that oppose the driving muscles and reduces the chances of injury to these opposing muscles. Third, it develops endurance in upper-body muscles that might otherwise fatigue in a long event and detract from the athlete's performance. Fourth, it builds strength in muscles that stabilize joints, thus reducing the possibility of injury.

Runners often express their reluctance to using weights for fear that they will add bulk or will slow down due to tight muscles (muscle-bound). Neither of these will happen to the majority of runners. Most people do not easily gain muscle mass and high-mileage runners seldom do. But, if some undesired muscle mass is added, the runner should eliminate the exercises that contributed to the hypertrophy, and through lack of use the muscle will atrophy. Muscle stiffness is overcome by stretching.

For the recreational or fitness runner, the benefits of strength training are even more obvious. Strengthening of some muscle groups helps to prevent injuries such as shinsplints, sprained ankles and knee pain. Avoiding injuries keeps the recreational runner on the road and away from the doctor. Also, since cardiovascular-respiratory endurance is only one part of fitness, a fitness program should include the other elements of fitness—namely flexibility and strength. Strength training and stretching are completely compatible with running, and the combination of the three make a great fitness program.

I run, stretch and strength train. Having the endurance, flexibility, and strength that I have developed over the past decade allows me to participate in a variety of other sports with little or no physical preparation. I might downhill ski or cross-country ski, or canoe or kayak on a weekend and have minimal or no soreness the next day. Also, since I have high levels of cardiovascular and muscle endurance, I can enjoy my weekend outings with less fatigue, and therefore less chance of injury, than others who do not train regularly.

John Jesse, coach and author, advocates strength training especially for muscle groups that have traditionally been neglected by runners: leg flexors (hamstrings), shoulder blade adductors (trapezius), abdominal and hip flexor muscles, ankle dorsi flexion (shin muscles), and trunk extensors (lower-back muscles). These groups are well-represented in the following recommendations.

Strength Programs for Sports 147

Sprints. Exercises for sprinters are used to develop strength and power. Do 8 - 10 repetitions of each exercise in each of three sets. To develop explosive running power, do rapid repetitions.

Exercise

Group	Motion	Exercises
1a	Leg extension	Stepups, leg extensions, leg press
1b	Leg flexion	Hamstring curls
2a	Hip extension	Swimmer's kick
2b	Hip flexion	Full situps, leg raises
4a	Trunk extension	Back extension
5a	Arm extension	Bench press, pushups, dips
5b	Arm flexion	Curls
6a	Arm abduction	Bent lateral raise
7a	Arm elevation	Upright row, military press, lateral dumbbell raise
7b	Arm depression	Lat pulldown
8a	Ankle extension	Calf raises
8b	Ankle flexion	Shin strengtheners, toe raises

Middle- and long-distance running. On long training runs the principal driving muscles of the legs get all the workout they need; however, other muscle groups do not get enough of a workout to develop increased strength, but they can fatigue. Strength training for the endurance runner is aimed at strengthening these other muscle groups. Build strength early in the offseason with 8 - 12 repetitions and then develop muscle endurance by doing 15 - 25 repetitions in either two or three sets. Aerobic strength training is ideal for distance runners, as it gives strength training benefits in an endurance format and it is a time-efficient method of strength training.

In the offseason add exercises for leg extension and flexion, hip flexion and ankle eversion. During the preseason or competitive season add the arm swing with dumbbells.

To do the arm swing exercise hold a pair of dumbbells with an overhand grip—that is so your thumbs face forward. Alternately swing the dumbbells, backward as far as possible and forward, up to eye level.

Exercise Group	Motion	Exercises
2a	Hip extension	Swimmer's kick
4a	Trunk extension	Back extension
4b	Trunk flexion	Abdominal curls
6a	Arm abduction	Bent row
6b	Arm adduction	Wide-grip bench press
7a	Arm elevation	Upright row, military press
7b	Arm depression	Lat pulldown
8b	Ankle flexion	Shin strengtheners, toe raises

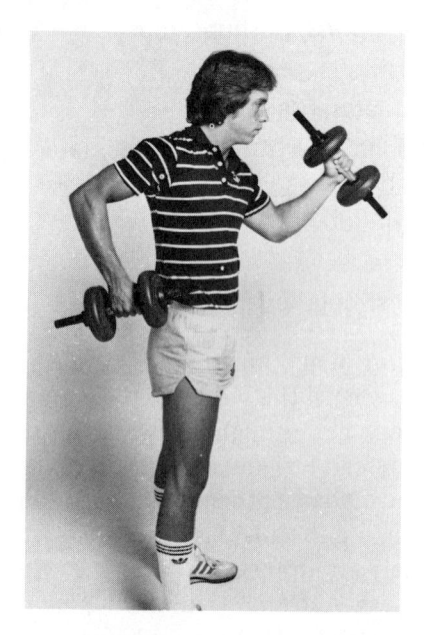

Dumbbell arm swing for running form.

SNOWSHOEING

Snowshoeing is no more than walking on snow with the aid of snowshoes. However, without some preparation for your first outing of the season your muscles will tire quickly. To prevent having a miserable day, train your cardiovascular system through activities like running. Also use weight training to improve strenght in these muscle groups:

- Leg Abductors—A wide foot stance is needed when wearing snowshoes and the hip abductors will fatigue early unless they have been conditioned.

- Hip flexors—In fresh powder you can sink 6-19 inches on every step. Strong hip flexors are needed to pull your leg out of your "post hole" and onto fresh snow.
- Ankle extensors (calf muscles)—These muscles will tire going uphill. Make sure that they are flexible as well as strong.
- Leg extensors—With one foot on fresh snow and the second sunk deep in the powder you need strength and endurance in the quadriceps to keep going.
- Ankle flexors (shin muscles)—This group comes into play when pulling the shoe upward with the toes pointing up.

The following exercises should be used for the preseason. They can be used in season during the week if you snowshoe only on weekends. In early preseason training try to develop muscle strength by doing 8 - 12 repetitions of each exercise. As the season draws near, concentrate more on muscle endurance and cardiovascular fitness. Increase the number of repetitions, to 15 - 25, decreasing the resistance if need be. Try doing these exercises as part of an aerobic strength-training program.

Exercise Group	Motion	Exercises
1a	Leg extension	Leg press, squats, leg extension
2b	Hip flexion	Full situps, double leg raise
3a	Leg abduction	Lateral leg raise
4a	Trunk extension	Back extension/hyperextension
4b	Trunk flexion	Abdominal curl, side bends
8a	Ankle extension	Calf raises
8b	Ankle flexion	Shin strengtheners, toe raises

SOCCER

This is a game whose outcome depends on skill and aerobic conditioning. However, strength can prepare the player during the offseason. Start by doing 8 - 12 repetitions in three sets. As the season approaches, work toward developing muscular endurance—by increasing the repetitions and by using an aerobic weight training program.

Exercise Group	Motion	Exercises
1a	Leg extension	Squats, leg press, leg extension
1b	Leg flexion	Hamstring curls
3a	Leg abduction	Lateral leg raise
3b	Leg adduction	Partner-assisted adduction
4a	Trunk extension	Back hyperextension
4b	Trunk flexion	Abdominal curls, side bends
6b	Arm adduction	Bent rows
7a	Arm elevation	Military press
8a	Ankle flexion	Shin strengtheners, toe raises
8c	Ankle eversion	Ankle roll overs
10a	Neck extension	Partner-assisted extension, 4-way neck machine
10b	Neck flexion	Partner-assisted flexion, 4-way neck machine

SWIMMING

It is a common misconception that weight training and swimming are incompatible. However, Dr. James E. Counsilman, renowned swimming coach of Indiana University and the U.S. Olympic team, has stated: "The use of heavy resistance exercises is now accepted practice for competitive swimmers." He uses weight training to develop strength in his swimmers because it is more efficient in terms of the available training hours. He does warn, however, that an overall strength-training program can be detrimental to a swimmer. This can occur if a swimmer gains mass in muscles that do not greatly contribute to his movement through the water. Thus, he advises swimmers to concentrate strength-training programs only on those muscles that propel the swimmer.

The swimmer should choose between an orientation of strength, few repetitions with a heavy load, or endurance, many repetitions with a lighter load. I suggest a strength-oriented program for off-season training. This will increase strength most efficiently. As the season draws near, the training program should switch to exercises that are closely similar to those used for a particular stroke. Equipment to accommodate such exercises is usually not available at health clubs or gyms and we have chosen not to include those exercises.

Many coaches now suggest using isokinetic instead of isotonic exercises. This is based on the theory that since swimming is an isokinetic exercise, a strength-training program should be isokinetic to be compatible. Unfortuately, lack of availability of isokinetic equipment may preclude a swimmer from following this advice.

Counsilman suggests exercises from six groups.

Exercise Group	Motion	Exercises
1a	Leg extensors	Leg extensions, leg press, squats
2a	Hip extension	Swimmer's kick with ankle weights
5a	Arm extension	Triceps press, bench press—wide grip to emphasize the pectorals in the chest and narrow grip to emphasize the triceps and arm extensors
7b	Arm depression	Lat pulldown, straight arm pulldown
8a	Ankle extension	Calf raise

Exercises of secondary importance are:

2b	Hip flexion	Double leg raise, full situps
4a	Trunk extension	Back hyperextension
4b	Trunk flexion	Abdominal curls, full situps

VOLLEYBALL

Volleyball requires leg strength for vertical jumping and maintaining the low squat position in the backcourt, and strength in the trunk flexors and extensors for spiking. Any extra body weight degrades leaping ability and is undesirable.

To build leaping ability a strength program built around the squats exercise is recommended. Start by doing squats with one half your body weight or less. Keep the weight constant and increase the repetitions up to 50 per set. Do two sets per workout. When you have reached 50 repetitions, increase the weight 10 - 20 pounds and start building up to 50 repetitions again. Do these motions at the same speed you would while playing a game. Slowly squat into a comfortable position. Then jump upward quickly, pushing up on the barbell with your hands.

In the offseason use weights that allow you to do 8 - 12 repetitions. During the preseason emphasize endurance by doing more repetitions.

Here are the exercises for a strength development program for volleyball. Except for the squats, do 8 - 12 repetitions.

Exercise Group	Motion	Exercises
1a	Leg extension	Squat
1b	Leg flexion	Hamstring curls
4a	Trunk extension	Back extension
4b	Trunk flexion	Abdominal curls, side bends
7a	Arm elevation	Military press
7b	Arm depression	Straight arm pulldown
8a	Ankle extension	Calf raise
8c	Ankle eversion	Ankle rolls
9b	Wrist flexion	Wrist curls

WRESTLING

Wrestlers need to have great aerobic and strength conditioning. In recommending an exercise program it is tempting to include all exercise groups. Train for strength in the offseason and endurance (15 - 25 repetitions) in the preseason.

Exercise Group	Motion	Exercises
1a	Leg extension	Leg press, squat, leg extension
2a	Hip extension	Swimmer's kick
4a	Trunk extension	Back hyperextension
4b	Trunk flexion	Abdominal curls
5a	Arm extension	Dips, bench press, pushups
5b	Arm flexion	Chinups, barbell curl
6a	Arm abduction	Bent rows
7a	Arm elevation	Upright rows, military press
9a	Wrist extension	Reverse wrist curls
9b	Wrist flexion	Wrist curls

CHART CONTD. NEXT PAGE.

CHART CONTD. FROM PREVIOUS PAGE.

Exercise Group	Motion	Exercises
10a	Neck extension	Partner-assisted, 4-way neck machine
10b	Neck flexion	Partner-assisted flexion, 4-way neck machine

7

Strength Programs for Fitness

....strength fitness is no longer the sole domain of youth. It is a highly prized possession that today's new "normal" middle-aged man takes pride in maintaining...." "Strength fitness is a....positive quality, and a vital life force."

—John O'Shea

Most popular fitness programs neglect any real development of muscle strength. Yet fitness is usually defined as a state of well-being which includes cardiovascular-respiratory endurance, muscle strength, flexibility, and coordination. A true fitness program should include all of these elements—including muscle toning.

The fitness benefits from strength training are numerous. There is a feeling of well-being having just done a hard workout. Muscles feel tight, but good. Besides this general good feeling, strength training can prevent, or in some cases, rehabilitate injuries. For example, the common complaint of lower backache can, in many cases, be relieved with stretching and strengthening. Strengthening the ankle muscles can help prevent sprains, and there are many other examples. Not that strength training is an elixir—but it can help. If you participate in physical activities, especially on a once-a-week schedule, strength training can make the activities more enjoyable, less fatiguing and less dangerous.

But in the final analysis no one keeps up a fitness training program solely for the reasons listed above. If you enjoy doing an activity you will continue it—if not, you will not continue it. Some people abhor lifting weights—they should try some other form of exercising. However, most people have not seriously tried weight training and would be surprised to find they might enjoy it. This is especially true for women.

Weight training is fun. If you already do aerobic workouts three or four days a week, strength training is great for the alternate days. It adds variety and balance to your fitness program. It also keeps you active, and aerobic strength training can maintain your cardiovascular fitness should an injury interrupt your other aerobic training. Although aerobic strength training is not as efficient in developing aerobic capacity as is running, it is still applicable for aerobics.

If you are not into aerobics, start a strength-training program. After a few weeks, try running, cycling, or swimming on the alternate days. These activities use more calories per minute than does strength training and they develop cardiovascular-respiratory fitness more rapidly and to a high degree. With the combination of strength, stretching, and aerobics workouts you will be fit.

GETTING STARTED

Here are a few suggestions for your first few workouts. Following them will make your entry into the weight room easier.

Plan your first workout. Write out an exercise schedule, listing in order the exercises you want to do. Leave room on the schedule to write in the weights you use and the number of repetitions you do for each set. See the example exercise plan here. Make sure you take your written notes and a pencil with you. Unless you are familar with the exercises you will undoubtedly forget which exercises you wanted to do or how many reps you did do. You will use repetition count as a guide for determining when you should increase or decrease the exercise resistance. These notes also serve as written history of your progress and filling in the circles for each workout can be a motivating factor in itself.

Here is a sample workout schedule to use. Write in the date at the top. You can also write in your body weight. However, if you do not work out at the same time of day, anomalous fluctuations in your weight will show up. List the exercises you want to do along the left margin. Eight exercises is a good number to start with. In the circles, record the weights used and the repetitions done for each set. I have divided the circles into three compartments, assuming you will do three sets.

Strength Programs for Fitness 157

DATE

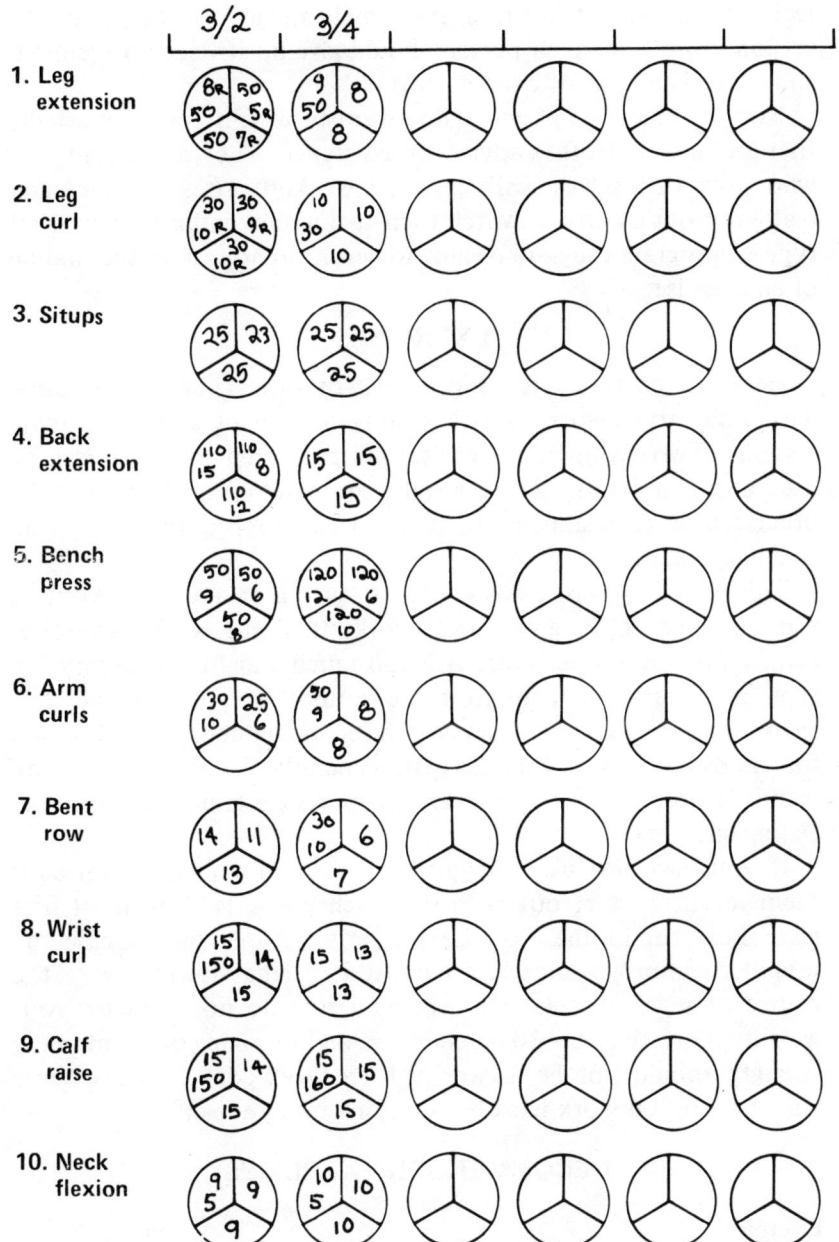

	3/2	3/4				
1. Leg extension	8R/50 / 50/5R / 50 7R	9/8 / 50 / 8				
2. Leg curl	30/30 / 10R/9R / 30/10R	10/10 / 30 / 10				
3. Situps	25/23 / 25	25/25 / 25				
4. Back extension	110/110 / 15/8 / 110/12	15/15 / 15				
5. Bench press	50/50 / 9/6 / 50/8	120/120 / 12/6 / 120/10				
6. Arm curls	30/25 / 10/6	50/8 / 9/8 / 8				
7. Bent row	14/11 / 13	30/6 / 10/7				
8. Wrist curl	15/14 / 150/15	15/13 / 13				
9. Calf raise	15/14 / 150/15	15/15 / 160/15				
10. Neck flexion	9/9 / 5/9	10/10 / 5/10				

If possible have a friend work out with you. This will make you feel more confident in the strange environment, and will make the session more fun. Each person should give positive reinforcement, and critical analysis of exercise form.

You will find that people who seriously weight train are usually friendly and will offer advice or assistance. They admire anyone who, like themselves, will show up workout after workout and really put out an effort. Watch their techniques and ask them what type of program they are doing; however, do not ask in the middle of an exercise.

EXERCISES

Here are exercises for a general workout. They can be done within the framework of either conventional or aerobic training sessions. Two groups of exercises are presented—one that can be used at a gymnasium where weight equipment is available and the other can be done almost any place, because it requires no specialized equipment.

This set of exercises was chosen to give a balanced workout. It was also chosen to give a safe workout. Some weight exercises can, if done improperly or with too much weight, cause injuries. It is much more difficult to injure yourself doing these exercises than doing some of the others often recommended. A third reason for choosing these is that they are generally the exercises recommended most often for the various sports programs (see the preceding chapter).

If you have not used weights before or if you have not used them recently, start out with very light weights. You must first learn how to do the exercise properly before you increase the weight to improve muscle tone. Add weight slowly—over the course of several weeks. As a general rule do not increase your weights more than 5 - 10 percent a week. Improving or maintaining strength should not be a two- or three-week goal. Improvements will come if you work hard but do not strain yourself.

RECOMMENDED EXERCISES

Exercise Group	Motion	Using Equipment	No Equipment
1a	Leg extension	Leg extension	Step-ups
1b	Leg flexion	Hamstring curls	Standing leg curl

CHART CONTD. NEXT PAGE.

CHART CONTD. FROM PREVIOUS PAGE.

Exercise Group	Motion	Using Equipment	No Equipment
2a	Hip extension	Swimmer's kick	Hip raise
4a	Trunk extension	Back extension	Toe touch
4b	Trunk flexion	Abdominal curl	Abdominal curl
5a	Arm extension	Bench press	Pushups
5b	Arm flexion	Curls	Narrow-grip chinups
6b	Arm adduction	Bent lateral raise	Partner resistance or chest expander
7a	Arm elevation	Military press	Lateral arm raise
7b	Arm depression	Lat pulldown	Wide grip chinups

After doing six weeks of these exercises change some of them. You could substitute other exercises from the same exercise groups (see Chapter 5) or substitute between exercise groups. Keep your program balanced between opposing muscle groups. You should not try to equalize the work done by each group since some muscles are inherently stronger than others. But do not continually exercise one member of an opposing pair without some work on the other member.

Modify your program to meet your needs and in response to your progress. If you mindlessly walk into the weight room and do the same old routine every workout, you are wasting your time (and probably getting bored). To make the workouts count, think before you lift.

After several months, when you have developed good form and you know what weights you need, try an aerobic strength-training workout. Aerobic strength training (AST) is ideal for a fitness program since it develops strength and aerobic fitness at the same time. As with any compromise, AST has limitations. Strength is developed at a slower rate than with conventional techniques—although only slightly slower. Also aerobic training effects are smaller than with a strictly aerobic exercise program—for example running. Nonetheless, AST is extremely time-efficient and gives training in both areas. For a complete fitness program I recommend AST plus some combination of aerobic exercises—running, swimming, or cycling.

8

Injuries

> *"It is well established that strengthening of the muscle surrounding body joints is an absolute must for the prevention of injuries."*
>
> —John Jesse

Strength training plays a more dominant role in preventing injuries than in causing them. In one survey of weight trainers, fewer than 2 percent of the respondents reported suffering an injury. On the other hand, strengthening exercises are recommended for preventing sports injuries and for rehabilitating injuries.

There are three principal benefits of injury prevention from strength improvements. First, strength training builds muscles and tendons. The stronger they are, the more stress they can bear. Thus muscular development of the extensors and flexors of the lower leg helps protect the ligament and cartilage of the knee.

Second, by developing strength you improve endurance. Many sports injuries occur late in a contest when the participant is tired. As fatigue increases and available muscle strength decreases, muscles are less able to take stress, action becomes less coordinated and injuries occur more frequently.

The development of muscle strength in the antagonist or opposition muscles is the third benefit. Since muscles cause movement only by pulling, not by pushing, every limb or body movement is controlled by at least two opposing muscles. For example, the triceps in the back of the upper arm extend the lower arm and the biceps flex the lower arm. These muscles oppose each other's action and are called an antagonistic pair.

In many sports, strength is employed in one muscle or muscle group. For instance, in sprinters strong quadriceps muscles (along the front of the thighs) are a must. These muscles straighten the lower leg and provide the power for running. The muscles that bend the leg at the knee, the hamstrings, often receive little strength training. The result is that the quadriceps are much stronger than the hamstring—this is called an imbalance between antagonists. Because the hamstrings are weak, they can be slow to relax. The sprinter drives the leg downward and the stronger quadriceps pulls on the weaker hamstring, possibly causing a muscle pull in the hamstrings. However, when the hamstrings are strengthened, they respond quicker and are less likely to be injured. One of the goals of any strength-training program should be to develop a good balance between the various pairs of antagonistic muscles. Programs that emphasize work on only one member of a pair can lead to injuries and poor posture.

A common example of a muscle imbalance is the development of the chest or pectoral muscles but not the trapezius muscles in the upper back. The muscles that bring arms together across the chest are strengthened by the bench press (or pushups) and lateral arm raises or flies. These are exercises commonly found in a workout. Less common are bent-back rows or reverse flies, which strengthen the muscles that pull the shoulder blades together and the arms back. The result of neglecting the exercises for the back is slumping shoulders, ill-fitting clothes and generally poor posture. When strength training, remember the laws of physics: for every action there is an equal and opposite reaction. If you train the action muscles, make sure you train their antagonists, the reaction muscles. The exercises listed in Chapter 5 are arranged in sets corresponding to antagonistic pairs. For example, quadriceps exercises are listed under 1a and hamstring exercises under 1b.

Weight training is often prescribed for rehabilitating injuries. Weight-training machines that limit motion to a particular direction allow controlled strength training. Being able to gradually increase the resistance of a rehabilitation exercise allows the patient to start with minimal resistance and work to his limit with little chance of reinjury. Strengthening the muscles also helps prevent further injury.

Injuries can occur, however, during a strength workout. Like many sport injuries, these can easily be prevented with care and common sense.

PREVENTION OF STRENGTH TRAINING INJURIES

The benefits of strength are achieved with regular workouts over a long period of time. Trying to get back in shape in one workout will be at the least, disappointing, and possibly injurious. Trying to keep to an unrealistic schedule of improvement, or worse yet, trying to compete with someone else is not sensible. You must be objective in assessing your ability and fitness; and choose exercise resistance, intensity and duration that are appropriate for you. If you are unsure of your strength, it is better to err by underestimating it rather than overestimating it. Choosing weights that are too light may result in an unproductive workout; but if you sustain an injury by using weights that are too heavy, you could miss several workouts. Thus the most important element in injury prevention is establishing and staying with a sensible workout plan.

To be effective, exercises must be done correctly. When done incorrectly they can cause injuries. The most common example is the squat exercise. Squats develop the driving muscles of the legs, the quadriceps. Since these muscles are important in all sports that require running or jumping, there is a great deal of interest in strengthening them. The squat or deep knee bend exercise can strengthen the quadriceps; however, knee injuries can be sustained by squatting too low, beyond an individual's limits of flexibility. Because of the danger to knees, many coaches do not recommend squats. However, if done properly, squats are a great exercise.

There are many other examples of doing an exercise incorrectly which leads to an injury. When doing supine lateral arm raises, elbows should be flexed slightly, not locked. This places the stress on the arm muscles and less on the elbow joint. Doing situps incorrectly can lead to back injuries. An even greater potential danger to the back is doing bent rows improperly. All of these exercises are safe—when done properly.

Just picking up a dumbbell or weight can hurt your back. Bending at the waist to pick up a heavy load places a huge stress on the muscles of the back. To find out how much stress there is, multiply the length of your back (say 1.5 feet) times the weight you are picking up. Thus, the torque on the back in this example is 1.5 foot pounds times the weight. For muscles that get little exercise in our "upright" society, this force can be large and very often too large. Weights that your back can handle when it is straight,

164 INJURIES

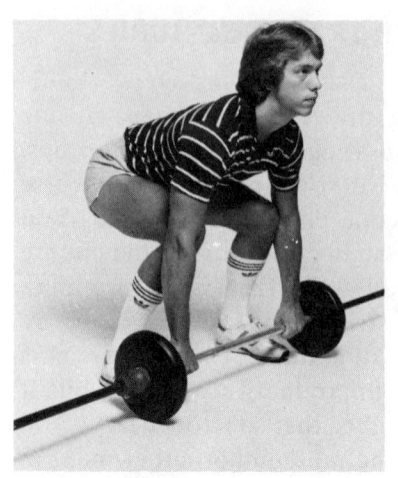

Right way: Knees bent, back straight.   Wrong way: knees straight, back bent.

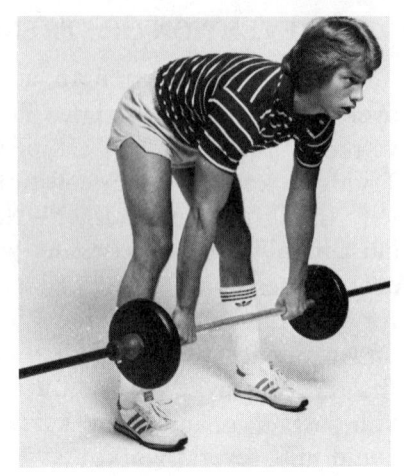

it may not be able to handle when it's bent. Bend your knees and hold your head upright when picking up weights.

Another aspect of doing exercises correctly is doing them slowly enough so that you are controlling the weights. When a barbell ceases to be level, there is the potential for losing control of the weights. This seldom occurs when the weights are being moved slowly. (Using weight machines eliminates this problem but robs you of natural or balanced strength development.) The only time that exercises should be done rapidly is in speed-or power-training programs. For these it is best to use weight machines.

Warm-up exercises are essential to prevent injuries. They should be done both before and after each strength workout. Before a workout, a full regime of stretches should be completed. Doing strengthening exercises correctly requires movement through the full range of motion, so it is important to stretch the muscles through their full range. Stretching should be done statically, not ballistically. That is, stretch positions should be held for 10 - 15 seconds. Bouncing to achieve greater stretches, the ballistic method, is less controlled and can lead to overstretching injuries. The correct stretch position is where a pleasant sensation is felt in the muscle. If normal breathing is interrupted or if pain is felt, the stretch has been carried too far.

After a bout of stretching I recommend going through the entire set of exercises with either very light weights or no weights.

While doing this, concentrate on achieving full extension and contraction and using good exercise form. Following this procedure will warn you of muscle soreness or injury. It has the secondary benefit of mentally and psychologically preparing you for the workout. You can review what you want to accomplish in the workout in terms of form, resistance and repetition, and you can psych yourself up to do a good workout.

Finally, you can do a minute or so of actual warming up. Muscles are most elastic when warm. A few jumping jacks or other fast movements are all that is required.

When the workout is finished, it should be followed by another round of stretching. Undoubtedly, a few muscles will be sore, and the stretching will make them feel better. It will reduce the tightness. Stretching after exercising is the first step in preparing for the next workout.

Environmental conditions are important in preventing injuries related to heat. Weight rooms are often poorly ventilated. They can become hot and humid—conditions that are not conducive to a good workout. If possible, keep the temperature in the high 60s and proper air circulation. Especially on warm days, interrupt the workout for a drink of water. If you are sweating, drink water even before you notice a thirst.

Many people hold to the old belief that you can sweat pounds off and they come to a workout wearing sweatsuits or even rubber suits. Sweating reduces body weight but as soon as you go to the drinking fountain, weight increases again. Losing water is not the equivalent of losing calories. If you do not replace the water lost by perspiration you can suffer from any one of several ailments, ranging from heatstroke to kidney failure. These are extremes, rarely encountered, but certainly your workout will suffer if you are dehydrated. Leave the extra clothing at home—or better yet do not buy it.

Wear comfortable, loose-fitting clothing. Wear shoes, because there are many objects in weight rooms to stub a toe on. T-shirts are necessary and even mandated by public health officials in some places. Beyond a T-shirt, shorts, shoes and socks, wear whatever you need to keep you warm, but not hot or sweaty.

Use common sense to prevent injuries. Before lifting a barbell, check the collars to make sure that they are securely fastened. Falling weights make a racket and possibly can lead to a broken toe or two. When doing bench presses or squats with a barbell,

166 INJURIES

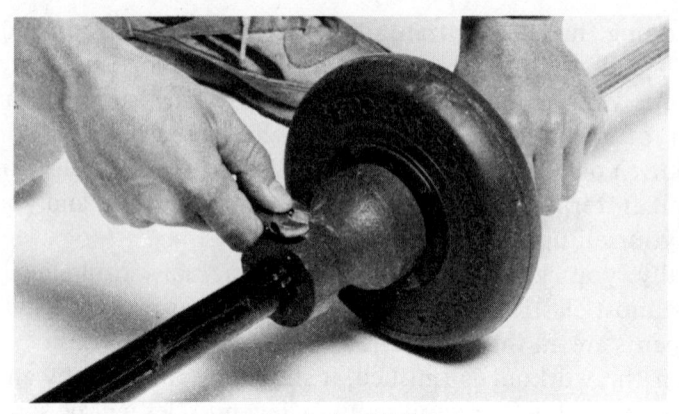

Make sure collars are secure on dumbbells.

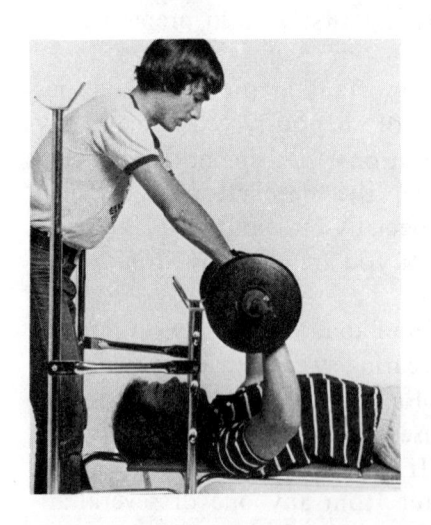

A spotter (or spotters) should be used for barbell bench press.

have a spotter assist you. That way you can work your muscles to fatigue and not worry about being pinned in place by an immovable barbell.

When tired or ill do not lift. Everyone suffers from a minor cold now and then, but only you can decide if you should work out in this condition. But for anything more serious than a cold, don't. Also, if you are going to do two workouts in a day, say running and strength training, do the strength training first. Either activity will suffer from being second, unless separated by several hours.

TREATMENT OF INJURIES

If an injury occurs during a workout, stop immediately and ascertain the seriousness of it. By not stopping, you can only make the injury worse. Often immediate attention to a minor injury will minimize the time lost to training, so the first step in the treatment of an injury is prevention of additional damage.

Often you can continue your workout by avoiding one or two exercises that work the injured muscle or joint, but even this is not highly recommended because further damage could occur. Also an injury often makes you lose timing and coordination as you unconsciously try to avoid pain in the injured part. This can lead to poor exercise form and even other injuries.

After stopping the workout, an aggressive first-aid procedure should be initiated. The emphasis here is on the word aggressive. The sooner something is done to minimize the damage of the injury, the sooner the injured part will heal. Watch what happens on the sidelines of a professional football game when a player's ankle is sprained. The trainers go to work immediately.

There are three typical injuries that occur in strength training: strains, sprains, and muscle soreness. For minor occurrences of these injuries home treatment will suffice. But for any case where there is doubt about the seriousness of the injury or when the home treatment does not bring rapid healing, don't delay seeing a physician.

Strains. Strains are tears or ruptures of muscle or tendon fibers They are commonly called muscle pulls. They occur when the force exerted on a muscle or tendon is greater than the strength of the fiber. In the example cited above, a sprinter with a hamstring-quadriceps muscle imbalance might suffer a hamstring pull or strain. The quadriceps are so much stronger that if the hamstring does not relax while the quadriceps are contracting, muscle fiber in the hamstring can be torn. Stretching and strengthening exercises are recommended for prevention of muscle pulls.

Very minor muscle strains can heal in a few days. More serious pulls may take four or five weeks to heal. In such cases, limited training can resume after two weeks provided it is at a low level of exertion. Gradually increase the intensity of the workout; pushing too hard or too fast will probably cause reinjury.

The body responds to strains and sprains in the same way: pain, swelling, discoloration and possible loss of movement of the injured part. This response is caused by the breaking of blood vessels in the muscle or tendon. Blood and other fluids flowing into the area cause the conditions listed.

First aid is to isolate and reduce the flow of fluids. Stopping the internal bleeding will minimize pain and swelling. Also, since the fluids must be removed before healing is completed, the smaller the quantities of fluid to start with, the faster the healing will occur.

To prevent further bleeding, apply ice as soon as possible. Immerse the injury in an ice bath or wrap an ice bag around it. If you do not have any ice bag, use a heavy-duty zip-lock plastic bag. Keep ice on the injury for 10 or 15 minutes. Longer applications do not cause further improvements and may injure the skin. Repeat this treatment every few hours for one or two days, following the injury.

Elevate the injury as well. This helps remove blood and other fluids from the site of the injury. Constrictive bandages can be applied after the ice treatment, to lessen the bleeding.

When the bleeding and fluid loss have completely stopped— usually that is 36-48 hours after the occurrence of the injury— procedures are changed. Now the objective is to increase circulation, to remove fluids and promote healing. Apply heat in the forms of heat packs or whirlpools. Gentle massage also helps. Be careful when applying heat. If you start heat therapy too early, you may increase fluid loss in the injury and add days to the recovery time. It's better to wait the full 48 hours and be sure the fluid loss has stopped, rather than speeding up the loss with heat. Continue using constrictive bandages.

If you want to use a drug, either to reduce pain or speed healing, use aspirin. It does both, its cheap and it's safe, which is more than can be said about other drugs that may achieve the same results.

Sprains. Sprains occur in dramatic sequence when a joint is subjected to a motion or force it cannot withstand—a basketball player comes down from a rebound attempt and lands on the side of his foot. The muscles that rotate the foot about the ankle cannot take that stress, and tendons and muscles rupture around the ankle joint.

The response for strains does equally well for sprains. Use ice, elevation and constriction, immediately. With very painful sprains consult a doctor, because fractures sometimes occur with sprains.

Muscle soreness. Muscle soreness usually signifies that the muscles got more of a workout than they were accustomed to. It can indicate which muscles had been overlooked in previous workouts. If you eliminate the exercise that caused soreness, the muscles will never strengthen and soreness will return the next time you do a similar exercise. You should use soreness as an indicator of what is weak and needs more work.

Until your next workout, however, there are three things you can do. First, gently stretch the sore muscle. Second, apply heat. This will relax the muscle and stimulate blood circulation to the area. Keep heat on the area for no longer than 30 minutes and do that several times a day. Third, have the sore muscle massaged.

9

Strength Training for Women

Women can be strong. They have muscles and the ability to strengthen those muscles. They have many reasons to be strong, considering their daily routines requiring them to lift everything from babies to furniture.

But women have been gaining strength by accident, not by desire. They have been snatching, dead lifting, and clean jerking weights for years. The weights used cannot be found in any weight room, but they have helped build strength.

Archaic attitudes held by society have kept women out of the weight room. They made entering a weight room as taboo for women as entering a men's locker room.

Fortunately, a few women have ventured into this male-dominated world. They have found that the room is not as discriminating as they feared. The weights are as heavy for women as they are for men and the trace of a sweaty workout lingers for both.

The benefits from weightlifting are not exclusive to men. Heavy objects become a little easier to lift for women who strength train. Back injuries and strains are reduced by strengthening back and shoulder muscles. Greater accomplishments in sports can be achieved if muscles necessary to perform the sports are strengthened. Fatty tissue can also be reduced by weight training.

Today's women learned prejudices against weightlifting early in life. Physical education programs in school never encouraged them to discover muscular-strength potential. When the boys were growing strong with chinups and pushups, the girls were learning to be graceful with square dancing. While boys were developing their muscles, girls were stretching to "we must increase our bust."

172 STRENGTH TRAINING FOR WOMEN

Thanks to changing laws and greater social awareness, sports have become equally available to women as they have been for men. Weightlifting is one previously male-dominated sport now open to women.

MYTHS

The myths surrounding women lifting weights must be dispelled. They are partly responsible for the low number of women in weight-training programs.

The most damaging myth of all is that women will build large and bulging muscles from weightlifting. Women imagine themselves becoming a female version of Arnold Schwarzenegger. But

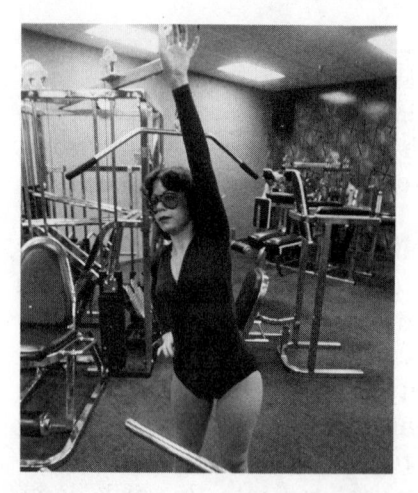

Women are entering weight rooms now.

women cannot build massive muscles because they have a low testosterone level, which is the hormone responsible for building muscle bulk. Studies show that most women develop only one-tenth the muscle mass of men who are the same size and follow the same weight-training program. Weight training was not recommended for women in the past because it was wrongly believed that women could not gain substantial muscular strength.

A well-known exercise physiologist, Dr. Jack Wilmore, ran a 10-week study to observe strength differences between men and women. Initially each subject lifted weights so that they could do only seven to nine repetitions. When the subjects were able to do 14 - 16 repetitions, more weight was added to bring the number of reps back down to the beginning number of seven to nine reps. The results showed that the muscular-strength difference between females and males depended on their unequal amounts of muscle mass.

Actually, most women have much more to gain through strength training than do men because they have never done it. They can make greater progress, in terms of relative strength improvement, than men can. Many female athletes report noticeable improvements in their performance after only a few weeks of strength training.

In our society, women are discouraged from lifting heavy objects. They are warned that this could badly injure them. The truth is that women can lift objects without injury if the proper techniques are used. They must learn to use the basic rules for weightlifting that men have been using for years. Some of these rules are outlined later in this chapter.

Another myth has been that women should not strength train during menstruation. This myth can be quickly shattered by pointing out that women have won Olympic gold medals and set world records during menstruation.

Some women who experience pain during menstruation even claim that exercising has eliminated the associated pain. This is not to say that every woman can reduce menstrual cramping, through exercise but it suggests that, at least for some women, exercise has helped.

HOW STRONG ARE YOU?

It is believed that overall strength can be closely determined by testing five muscle groups: leg extensors, hip flexors, knee extensors, forearms and elbow flexors. Here are a few simple tests to determine how strong you are right now. Keep in mind that these tests cannot give you an exact measurement of strength. They are designed to give you a point of reference for future comparisons.

Take these tests again after three weeks of training. Compare the results to see if you progressed.

BATHROOM SCALE SQUEEZE

Hold a bathroom scale in both hands with your thumbs on top and your fingers wrapped around in back. The dial should be facing you so that you can read the number of pounds squeezed. Stretch both arms out in front of you at shoulder-height and squeeze. Hold your grip for a few seconds and then record the number.

An average strength is 70 pounds. The stronger the grip, the more pounds you will be able to squeeze.

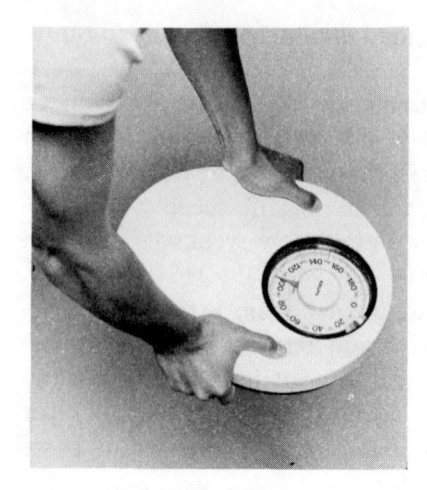

Bathroom scale squeeze measures your progress.

PUSHUP TEST

Women who are in good physical condition should be able to do at least five pushups.

A woman's upper body strength is less a man's, although lower body strengths are much more comparable. Many women will find the pushup test difficult, but after a few weeks of weight-lifting you will see a great improvement when you repeat this test.

Traditionally, women have been taught bent-knee pushups. In this pushup, you rest your lower body on your knees and not on your toes. If you prefer "modified pushups," do them. But you will limit your strength gain by using this easier pushup.

WALL SQUAT TEST

This test will evaluate your leg strength. You will need a watch or to be in a position to see the second hand of a clock.

Lean your back against a wall and slide down until you are in a sitting position, held up only by the pressure of your back against the wall and your legs. Your thighs should be horizontal and your feet flat on the floor. Be sure that your feet are a comfortable distance apart and that they are only about 12 to 14 inches away from the wall. Time how long you are able to maintain this position. Holding for a half-minute in this position is pretty good to start.

RULES FOR THE WEIGHT ROOM

Before you begin any of the programs suggested, read the following pointers.

- *Stretch.* With any exercise program you must first stretch. Use the stretching exercises described in Chapter 5.
- *Breathe properly.* For those who have never lifted weights, it is important to remember to breathe out when lifting weights, breathe in when lowering weights. Never hold your breath.
- *Choose proper weights.* When trying to determine what weight to use, choose one that will tax you. You should be able to complete the required reps (use 8 - 12 to start), but only by putting out a good deal of effort. If you reach the repetition goal for an exercise and feel you can do several more reps, do them.
- *Plateau effect.* During your training you may experience periods when you are unable to increase weight for a period of time. Do not be discouraged; this is a common occurrence, known as the plateau effect.
- *Lift weights properly.* Be careful when lifting with your back muscles. When lifting weights off the floor, bend your knees, keep your back straight, head up, and allow your leg muscles to do the work.
- *Medical examination.* If you are elderly, or you are leading a physically inactive life, a stress test using an EKG monitoring is advised before you start any exercise program. All women should seek their doctor's advise regarding strength training.

BEGINNING A STRENGTH PROGRAM

Many people begin exercise programs with great vigor, but find that their enthusiasm dwindles after a few weeks. Consider the following points before beginning your program:

1) How much time do you have to spend on strength training during the week?
2) What program will provide enough new challenges to keep you training?
3) How strong would you like to be?
4) Do you need to train with a group to give you the incentive to work out or do you want to work out alone?

Set your own strength goals and follow your own program.

All exercises listed in this chapter can be performed in a weight room or at home, with slight variations. If possible, try finding a gym with a weight room. Meeting others at a gym for a workout can mean the difference between whether you make strength training a way of life or a one-time thing.

Progressive overloading is used for the two types of programs suggested in this chapter. It makes the muscles work harder than usual by adding more and more weight over a period of time. When the program calls for more weight, try adding 2½ pounds.

Workouts should be at least three times a week, such as Monday, Wednesday, and Friday. As you progress in your strength training program, you can devise your own exercises and routines.

PROGRESSIVE REP SYSTEM

This program can take as little as 10 minutes for a workout. If you are pressed for time, this is for you.

Begin by using the initial reps and initial weight amounts, as listed on the accompanying exercise chart. Do one full set without resting between exercises. At each subsequent workout continue doing one set, but add one rep to each exercise. Decrease the weight suggested if you were unable to complete the advised number of reps. If it was too easy to complete the reps, add more weight.

Once the maximum rep amount (see exercise chart) is reached, test to see if you are ready for more weight. When you can lift a weight the maximum number of reps, then you are ready to add weight. You may find you can add weight to some exercises but not to others. This is fine; you do not have to increase the weight for all exercises at the same time.

If you decide that you can add more weight, drop back to the initial rep amount and continue doing one set of exercises with this weight.

Build back up to the maximum number of reps, and as before, test to see if more weight can be added. If you can, add more weight and drop back to the initial rep count. Continue this routine until you have reached your strength goal.

PROGRESSIVE SET SYSTEM

If you are able to spend more time, say 15 to 25 minutes three times a week on strength training, this program will develop your strength faster than the progressive rep system. As with the previous program, begin with the suggested initial rep and weight amount. Increase reps until you reach the maximum rep count. Then decide if additional weight can be added. If you can add weight, drop back to initial rep and weights and add another set of exercises instead of increasing the weight. If adding reps at each workout is too difficult, try adding them every other workout, or once a week.

When you have reached two sets of exercises with maximum reps, you have two options. You can either continue with two sets of exercises and increase your weights or you can drop back to initial reps and add a third set.

I suggest that you limit yourself to a maximum of three sets. When you reach three sets and maximum reps, begin adding weight.

Once you have reached your desired strength goal, continue with this weight amount. It is hoped that you will reach the goals set in the beginning and continue to improve.

EXERCISES

Exercise	Initial Reps	Maximum Reps	Muscle Group	Initial Weight Amount
Situp	12	16	Abdomen	No weight
Bench press	8	12	Pectorals, triceps	40 lbs.
Arm curls	8	12	Biceps	5 lbs/hand (dumbbells)
Stepups	12	16	Thigh	No weight
Calf raise	12	16	Calf	No weight
Arm Raise	8	12	Deltoids	5 lbs/hand
Hip extension	12	16	Buttocks	No weight
Back extension	12	16	Lower back	No weight
Wrist curls	8	12	Forearms	10 lbs.

EXERCISE CHART

Situp—Lie on your back, knees bent. With hands clasped behind your head, raise up toward your knees. To increase the resistance of this exercise, hold a weight behind your head.

Bench press—Lie on your back on a bench. Bend your knees and place your feet flat on the bench. This position helps keep you from using your back to lift the weights. Push the weights above your chest until your arms are fully extended, then lower them, and lift again. Do not let the weights return to a resting position until you have finished.

Arm curls — Stand with dumbbells in each hand with your palms facing forward. Keeping the upper part of your arm still, bring the weights up to meet your shoulders. Make sure your wrists do not bend. Slowly lower the weights to the beginning position—do not let them just drop down.

Hamstring curls—Hold onto something sturdy. Bend your leg and bring your foot up to touch your buttocks. Do not point your toes. If you are working out in a weight room, you can use a weight machine designed specifically for this exercise. Otherwise, increase resistance by using ankle weights.

Stepups—Place one foot on a step, then bring your other foot up beside it. Step back down with the second foot, followed again by the first. This full cycle is considered one rep. You may hold weights in your hands or attach ankle weights to increase resistance with this exercise. Do all the reps with one leg leading before you start with the other leg leading.

Calf raise—Stand with your heels hanging over the edge of a 2-by-4, or a step. Raise up on your toes, then lower your foot as low as is comfortable and then return to a level position. This is one rep. You may hold weights in your hands or attach ankle weights to increase resistance in this exercise.

Arm raise—Stand with your arms down at your sides, holding dumbbells in each hand. Keeping arms straight, raise both arms out to the side until they are at shoulder level. Be sure that your palms are facing down. Lower your arms slowly back to your sides.

Hip extension—Hold onto something sturdy. Keeping your leg and back straight, raise one leg backward and up as far as possible. Then bring it down. Continue raising and lowering the same leg until the reps have been completed. Then raise and lower the other leg. Ankle weights may be used to increase weight.

Leg extension—On your hands and knees, bring one knee up to meet your chest. Then extend this leg straight out behind you and lift your head up so that you are facing forward. Continue tucking and straightening the same leg until the number of suggested reps have been completed. Do the same for the other leg. Ankle weights may be used to increase resistance.

Wrist curls—Hold weights in both hands, palms up. Resting your forearms on your lap, raise and lower the weights by moving only your wrists. Allow the weights to drop over your knees so that your wrists can extend downward as far as possible. You may use a barbell or a pair of dumbbells for this exercise.

STRENGTH TRAINING AT HOME

For those of you who are going to work out at home and do not have weights available, here are some items you can use:

Long-handle broom. Place a broom handle through the handles of two bleach bottles (you add liquid in them for weight). Balance the bottles on either end and do wrist curls.

Two plastic one-gallon bleach bottles or milk bottles filled with water (eight pounds per bottle). Hold the bottles in either hand to do stepups and calf raises. Also, use them for wrist curls as described above.

Two half-gallon milk cartons, filled with dirt and top taped closed (six pounds per carton). These can be held in either hand to add weight for situps, arm curls, stepups, calf raises, arm raises and wrist curls.

Iron (two pounds). Lift by the handle and use in situps. You will need two irons if you use them for arm curls, stepups, calf raises, and arm raises.

Two-leg weights (homemade weights are described in Chapter 5). They can be attached to either legs or arms, to do hamstring curls, stepups, calf raises, arm raises, leg raises, and leg extensions.

If possible, purchase some five-pound dumbbells. They are easy to handle, which helps in doing the exercises correctly.

All the exercises listed here can be done in the home, except the bench press. Replace this with pushups or with an overhead weight drop.

Overhead weight drop works the triceps. Using both hands, hold a weight over your head. Bend your elbows, allowing the weight to drop behind your head. Then bring it back up over your head. This is one rep.

There are disadvantages to working with weights made from household items. The items that weigh enough to overload and build strong muscles are sometimes unmanageable. If you are trying to follow the suggested 2½-pound increase in weight, this exact amount might be hard to find.

PREGNANT AND STRONG

Luckily, pregnant women are no longer shut away behind closed doors for nine months. They can be physically active without harming the fetus. Pregnancy is a time of excitement and constant change. It is a time when food, exercise, and practically everything else is rated either good or bad for mom and baby.

If you are pregnant, now is not the time to start training for a strength contest. Of course, that does not imply that you cannot begin a strength program now. The earlier in the pregnancy you begin your strength program, the better. Ideally you should begin training before you become pregnant.

First, check with your doctor and explain the type of program you wish to start. He will probably tell you to do what feels good. Common sense is a big part of taking care of your body, whether you are pregnant or not.

There are a few uncomfortable side effects during pregnancy, but do not be alarmed or let them prevent you from exercising. Though some will show up no matter what you do, there are a few things you can do to make yourself more comfortable.

Varicose veins are common, but increased muscular activity stimulates the flow of blood back to the heart, helping to prevent the veins from dilating.

Very few pregnant women are free of backaches sometime. Relief can be obtained, though, by strengthening your lower back muscles and your stomach muscles.

Good posture becomes a must during pregnancy. Avoid slouching in chairs, even though it is a temptation. It is easier to get up from a chair in which you have been sitting straight, than one in which you have allowed yourself to slouch. After the seventh or eighth month, it takes only one time of having to ask for help out of a chair to remind yourself of this.

Hemorrhoids are most frequent toward the end of the pregnancy or after delivery. Instead of taking medication, try increasing your fluid, fruit, and fiber intake.

Leg cramps can be reduced by not pointing your toes. If your leg does cramp, pull your toes back toward you as far as possible and hold them there until the cramping subsides. Keeping your calf muscles strong and flexible will help limit calf cramps. Do the calf stretches shown in Chapter 5.

Each pregnancy is different for each woman; however, recent data suggests that the stronger, more active woman is better prepared to handle the last stages of childbirth. Proper breathing during childbirth is also important, and will be second nature if you have incorporated it in your strength program.

Most exercises recommended here can be done while pregnant. If any seem too difficult, modify them by reducing the weights or choosing other exercises that work the same muscle group.

The change in the center of gravity after the fourth month of pregnancy makes balancing more difficult, but this does not affect your strength. Follow all the weightlifting rules outlined in this chapter and you will enjoy an active pregnancy.

MODIFICATION OF EXERCISES DURING PREGNANCY

Situps—If using a slant board, you may find that a horizontal level is most comfortable. Instead of rising to a sitting position, raise just your head and shoulders. This modified situp still works the stomach muscles, which need strengthening now.

Pushups—These may be difficult to do after the fourth month, but arm and shoulder muscles will need to be strong. After childbirth, carrying your baby along with a bag filled with bottles, diapers, and toys will require considerable arm strength.

Instead of pushups, use the bench press. Be sure to bend your legs while lying on the bench. When getting up from the prone position, roll to one side before standing up. Do not get up by pulling yourself straight up. The overhead weight drop is also a good exercise to do if the bench press is not available.

ADDITIONAL EXERCISES

Kegels—This exercise is for the muscles of the pelvic floor, which are attached at the front and back of the pelvis. As the baby grows during pregnancy, this muscle is stretched. During delivery the muscle is stretched even more.

Kegels help keep the pelvic floor muscles toned. To know that you are doing a kegel properly, pretend that you are trying to stop the flow of urine. The muscles you tighten are the ones you want to strengthen. Contract the muscles for five seconds and then relax; this is one kegel. Kegels can be done anytime, anywhere, without anyone noticing. Pick a particular time of day or event that will remind you to kegel. Do about 50 kegels a day.

Pelvic tilt—This can be done lying on your back on the floor, on hands and knees or standing. To get the feel of what muscles to use, first lie on your back. With bent knees, push the small of your back down to the floor. Use this same muscle action while on your hands and knees. Once you know how pelvic tilts feel, you can do them standing.

Back raise—The importance of toning both stomach muscles

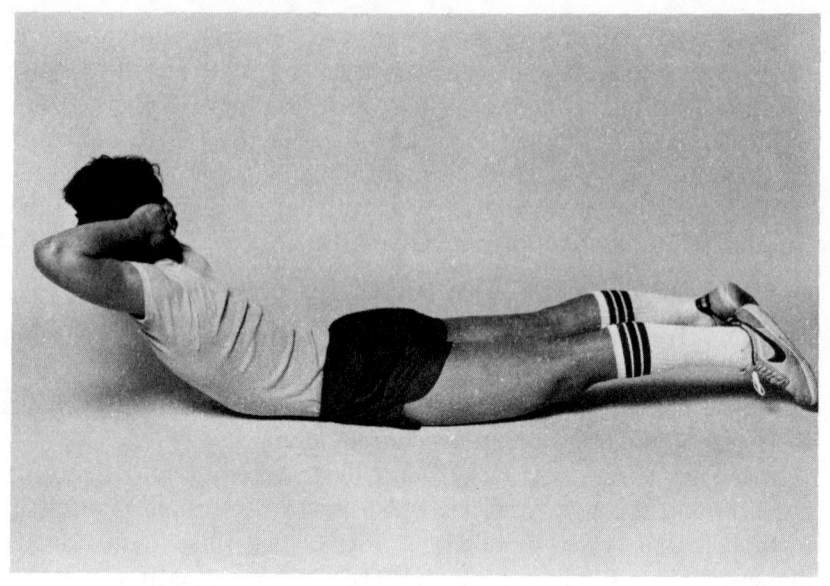

Arching the back while on stomach.

and back muscles during pregnancy cannot be stressed enough. Here is another good exercise, especially if you are having some backaches.

Relax, lying on the floor on your back. Raise your bottom up off the floor and arch your back. Your weight should be primarily resting on your legs and shoulders. Then lower yourself. Remember, roll onto your side to get off the floor when finished with this exercise.

POST DELIVERY

The sooner you become active after giving birth, the sooner you will feel normal. It is possible to resume some activity in the weight room a couple of weeks following delivery. Those who have had a cesarean may need to wait longer; and those who have had an episiotomy may find some exercises uncomfortable.

Having a baby is a very good experience, but it takes work. After the first week it is not uncommon to feel weak. A slow, short walk, even as short as a half block, helps. Begin exercising as soon as your doctor gives his approval. Go a little farther each day. Hours after delivery you can begin doing kegels.

A strength training program should fit your lifestyle. Whether you choose one for overall fitness or for a particular sport, it should be one you will continue doing. The more convenient and enjoyable the program, the longer it will be used.

Bibliography

Anderson, B. *Stretching*. P.O. Box 2734, Fullerton, CA: 1975.

Brady, M. Michael, and Lorns O. Skjemstad. *Ski Cross Country*. The Dial Press, 1974

Counsilman, J.E. *The Science of Swimming*. Englewood Cliffs, NJ: Prentice-Hall, 1968.

deVries, H.A. *Physiology of Exercise for Physical Education and Athletics*. Dubuque, IA: William C. Brown Publishers, 1966.

Dickinson, Art. "Medical Advice." *Nordic World*, Sept. - Oct. - Nov., 1979.

Gettman, L.R., and M.L. Pollock. "Circuit Weight Training: A Critical Review of Its Physiological Benefits." *The Physician and Sports Medicine,* January, 1981. Vol. 9, No. 1.

Hellebrandt, F.A., and S.J. Horitz. "Mechanisms of Muscle Training in Man: Experimental Demonstration of the Overload Principle." *The Physical Therapy Review,* 1956. Vol. 36, No. 6.

Hinson, Marilyn M. *Kinesiology*. Dubuque, IA: William C. Brown Publishers, 1977.

Jesse, John. *Strength, Power and Muscular Endurance for Runners and Hurdlers*. Pasadena, CA: The Athletic Press, 1971.

Keyes, Michael J. "Weight Lifting for the Pistol Shooter." *The American Marksman*. January, 1981.

Matthews, D.K., and E.L. Fox. *The Physiological Basis of Physical Education and Athletics*. W.B. Saunders Co. 1976.

Miller, Carl. *How to Use Weight Training For Your Specific Sport*. Sante Fe, NM: 1980.

O'Shea, John Patrick. *Scientific Principles and Methods of Strength Fitness.* 2nd ed. Addison-Wesley, 1976.

Prater, Gene. *Snowshoeing.* The Mountaineers. Seattle, WA: 1974

Reynolds, Bill. *Complete Weight Training Book.* Mountain View, CA: World Publications, 1976.

Ryan, A.J. "Sports Medicine Today." *Science,* Vol. 200; May, 1978.

Sobey, Ed. "Circuit Training." *Down River.* May, 1977.

Sobey, Ed. *The Complete Circuit Training Guide.* Mountain View, CA: Anderson World Inc., 1980.

Sorani, Robert. *Circuit Training.* Dubuque, IA: William C. Brown Co., 1966.

Weldon, G. *Weight Training for Women's Team Sports.* Weldon Publishing, 1977.

About the Author

Edwin Sobey is director of the Science Museum and Planetarium of Palm Beach County in West Palm Beach, Fla. Ed started running in 1966 as the result of a food fight in college. "Losing a foot race with a 240-pound lineman was the incentive I needed," he said. He's been using weights in his running program since 1976, and has found that they are a tremendous help in building strength without bulk. That same year Ed and his wife sailed a 54-foot ketch across the Pacific Ocean Ed has a Ph. D. in oceanography.

Recommended Reading

The following books, also available from Anderson World, can augment your exercise and fitness program. They are available from major bookstores or can be ordered directly from the publisher (1400 Stierlin Road, Mountain View, CA 94043).

THE RUNNER'S WORLD YOGA BOOK by Jean Couch with Nell Weaver. An easy-to-follow guide to using the principles of yoga for stretching, strengthening, and toning the body, and a good book to graduate to after making the initial commitment to embark on a fitness and health program. Paperback. $9.95.

THE RUNNER'S WORLD INDOOR EXERCISE BOOK by Richard Benyo and Rhonda Provost. A simple-to-understand guide to fitness and the exercising body, and how it responds to beginning exercise programs, with programs keyed to the beginner and oriented toward getting started comfortably indoors before moving into outdoor fitness training and outdoor sports. Paperback. $9.95.

THE RUNNER'S WORLD NATURAL FOODS COOKBOOK by Pamela Hannan. An easy-to-follow guide to recipes without sugar, with special attention to the vitamins that can be received from properly prepared food. Extensive recipes in a variety of categories. Spiral bound. $11.95.

THE RUNNER'S WORLD WEIGHT CONTROL BOOK by Michael Nash. A logical, realistic approach to losing weight and keeping it off forever that ignores the fad diets and gets right to the root of the problem: one's own image of self. A complete course in getting away from the multi-course meal. Paperback. $9.95.

DANCE AEROBICS by Maxine Polley. The rage that has swept the nation. Getting in shape and staying there through an ambitious program of enjoyable, fast-moving dance that builds aerobic fitness while toning muscles and doing away with unwanted weight. Quality paperback. $5.95.

GETTING YOUR EXECUTIVES FIT by Don T. Jacobs, Ph.D. The book that America's corporations have been waiting for. A book that, in one package, reviews all available information on corporate fitness, while making the information accessible to everyone from hourly worker to chairman of the board. Large format paperback. $12.95.